AF821055

ORL

Journal for Oto-Rhino-Laryngology and Its Related Specialties

Founded 1938 as 'Practica Oto-Rhino-Laryngologica' by J. Berberich and E. Schlittler, continued by L. Rüedi 1947–1970, E. Huizinga 1948–1970, C.R. Pfaltz 1968–1984

Managing Editor

W. Arnold, München

Editors

M. Anniko, Uppsala
P. van den Broek, Nijmegen
A. Ferlito, Udine
I. Friedmann, Stanmore
J.P. Harris, San Diego, Calif.
R. Häusler, Bern
K.-B. Hüttenbrink, Dresden
M. Igarashi, Tokyo
I. Kaufman Arenberg, Denver, Colo.
W. Lehmann, Genève
D.J. Lim, Los Angeles, Calif.
V.J. Lund, London
P. Montandon, Genève
R. Probst, Basel
O. Ribári, Budapest
R. Ruben, Bronx, N.Y.
W.F. Thumfart, Innsbruck
M. Tos, Copenhagen
C.D.A. Verwoerd, Rotterdam
T.J. Yoo, Memphis, Tenn.

Co-Editors

B.R. Alford, Houston, Tex.
H.-J. Altermatt, Bern
H.H. Birdsall, Houston, Tex.
K. Ehrenberger, Wien
D. Felix, Bern
H. Felix, Zürich
E. Ferekidis, Athens
U. Ganzer, Düsseldorf
J.-O. Gebbers, Luzern
J.P. Guyot, Genève
D.F.N. Harrison, London
S. Iurato, Bari
T. Janssen, München
R. Kau, München
W. Mann, Mainz
J. Nadol, Jr., Boston, Mass.
W.J. Oosterveld, Amsterdam
H. Rask-Andersen, Uppsala
M. Sanna, Piacenza
H. Stammberger, Graz
J.-I. Suzuki, Tokyo
G.A. Tavartkiladze, Moscow
T. Yamashita, Osaka
P. Zbären, Bern
H.P. Zenner, Tübingen

KARGER

Printed in Switzerland on acid-free paper by Reinhardt Druck, Basel

Appears bimonthly: 1 volume per year (6 issues)

Guidelines for Authors

ORL

Submission

Only original papers written in English are considered and should be sent to:

Prof. Dr. W. Arnold
S. Karger AG
Editorial Office ORL
P.O. Box
CH–4009 Basel (Switzerland)
Telephone +41 61 306 1357
Fax +41 61 306 1434
E-mail l.haas@karger.ch

Mailing address for courier deliveries only:
Allschwilerstr. 10
CH–4055 Basel (Switzerland)

Contributions for the section *Pathology Spot* (max. 10 manuscript pages, including tables, illustrations and references) should be sent to:

Prof. Alfio Ferlito
Department of Otolaryngology-Head and Neck Surgery
University of Udine
Policlinico Città di Udine
Viale Venezia 410
I–33100 Udine (Italy)
Telephone +39 0432 239302
Fax +39 0432 532179
E-mail a.ferlito@dsc.uniud.it

Manuscripts should be submitted in triplicate (with three sets of illustrations of which one is an original), typewritten double-spaced on one side of the paper, with a wide margin.

Conditions

All manuscripts are subject to editorial review. Manuscripts are received with the explicit understanding that they are not under simultaneous consideration by any other publication. Submission of an article for publication implies the transfer of the copyright from the author to the publisher upon acceptance. Accepted papers become the permanent property of 'ORL' and may not be reproduced by any means, in whole or in part, without the written consent of the publisher. It is the author's responsibility to obtain permission to reproduce illustrations, tables, etc. from other publications.

Arrangement

Title page: The first page of each paper should indicate the title (main title underlined), the authors' names, and the institute where the work was conducted. A short title for use as running head as well as the full address of the author to whom correspondence should be sent are also required.

Full address: The exact postal address complete with postal code must be given at the bottom of the title page. Please also supply phone and fax numbers, as well as your e-mail address.

Key words: For indexing purposes, a list of 3–10 key words in English is essential.

Abstract: Each paper needs an abstract of up to 10 lines.

Small type: Paragraphs which can or must be set in smaller type (case histories, test methods, etc.) should be indicated with a 'p' (petit) in the margin on the left-hand side.

Footnotes: Avoid footnotes. When essential, they are numbered consecutively and typed at the foot of the appropriate page.

Tables and illustrations: Tables and illustrations (both numbered in Arabic numerals) should be prepared on separate sheets. Tables require a heading and figures a legend, also prepared on a separate sheet. For the reproduction of illustrations, only good drawings and original photographs can be accepted; negatives or photocopies cannot be used. Due to technical reasons, figures with a screen background should not be submitted. When possible, group several illustrations on one block for reproduction (max. size 181 × 223 mm) or provide crop marks. On the back of each illustration, indicate its number, the author's name, and 'top' with a soft pencil.

Color illustrations: Up to 6 color illustrations per page can be integrated with the text at the reduced price of CHF 660.– / USD 545.00 per page. Color illustrations are reproduced at the author's expense.

References: In the text identify references by Arabic numerals [in square brackets]. Material submitted for publication but not yet accepted should be noted as 'unpublished data' and not be included in the reference list. The list of references should include only those publications which are cited in the text. Do not alphabetize; number references in the order in which they are first mentioned in the text. The surnames of the authors followed by initials should be given. There should be no punctuation other than a comma to separate the authors. Cite all authors, 'et al' is not sufficient. Abbreviate journal names according to the Index Medicus system. (Also see International Committee of Medical Journal Editors: Uniform requirements for manuscripts submitted to biomedical journals. N Engl J Med 1997;336:309–315.)

Examples
(a) Papers published in periodicals: Sun J, Koto H, Chung KF: Interaction of ozone and allergen challenges on bronchial responsiveness and inflammation in sensitised guinea pigs. Int Arch Allergy Immunol 1997;112:191–195.
(b) Monographs: Matthews DE, Farewell VT: Using and Understanding Medical Statistics, ed 3, revised. Basel, Karger, 1996.
(c) Edited books: Parren PWHI, Burton DR: Antibodies against HIV-1 from phage display libraries: Mapping of an immune response and progress towards antiviral immunotherapy; in Capra JD (ed): Antibody Engineering. Chem Immunol. Basel, Karger, 1997, vol 65, pp 18–56.

Page charges

There is no page charge for papers of 3 or fewer printed pages (including tables, illustrations and references). Each additional complete or partial page is charged to the author at CHF 650.– / USD 540.00. The allotted size of a paper is equal to approx. 8 manuscript pages (including tables, illustrations and references).

Galley proofs

Unless indicated otherwise, galley proofs are sent to the first-named author and should be returned with the least possible delay. Alterations made in galley proofs, other than the correction of printer's errors, are charged to the author. No page proofs are supplied.

Reprints

Order forms and a price list are sent with the galley proofs. Orders submitted after the issue is printed are subject to considerably higher prices.

KARGER

Fax + 41 61 306 12 34
E-Mail karger@karger.ch
www.karger.com

© 1999 S. Karger AG, Basel

The Guidelines for Authors are available at:
www.karger.com/journals/orl/orl_gl.htm

ORL

General Information

Publication data: 'ORL' is published 6 times a year. Volume 61 with 6 issues appears in 1999.

Subscription rates: Subscriptions run for a full calendar year. Prices are given per volume.

Personal subscription:
Subscription + postage and handling
CHF 348.50 + CHF 23.50 Europe
CHF 348.50 + CHF 35.50 Overseas
USD 266.50 + USD 23.50
(Must be in the name of, billed to, and paid by an individual. Order must be marked 'personal subscription'.)

Institutional subscription:
Subscription + postage and handling
CHF 697.– + CHF 29.40 Europe
CHF 697.– + CHF 44.40 Overseas
USD 533.00 + USD 29.40

Airmail postage: CHF 36.–, USD 30.00. (Extra per volume.)

Discount subscription prices:
Gesellschaft Schweizerischer HNO-Ärzte and Netherlands' Society of Otorhinolaryngology.

Microforms: Please direct all enquiries and orders to: University Microfilms Inc.
300 North Zeeb Road, P.O. Box 1346
Ann Arbor, MI 48106-1346 (USA)

Subscription orders: Orders can be placed at agencies, bookstores, directly with the Publisher
S. Karger AG, P.O. Box,
CH–4009 Basel (Switzerland)
or with any of the following distributors:
Deutschland: S. Karger GmbH, Postfach
D–79095 Freiburg
France: Librairie Luginbühl
36, bd de Latour-Maubourg, F–75007 Paris
Great Britain, Ireland: S. Karger Publishers
58 Grove Hill Road
Tunbridge Wells, Kent TN1 1SP
USA: S. Karger Publishers, Inc.
26 West Avon Road, P.O. Box 529
Farmington, CT 06085
India, Bangladesh, Sri Lanka:
S. Karger India Subscription Agency
B–5/132 Safdarjung Enclave
New Delhi-110029
Japan: Katakura Libri, Inc.
2F, Marushima Bldg, 4-6-17, Yushima,
Bunkyo-ku, Tokyo 113-0034

Change of address: Both old and new address should be sent to the subscription source.

Single issues and back volumes: Information can be obtained through the Publisher.

Advertising: Correspondence and rate requests should be addressed to the Publisher.

Book Reviews: Books are accepted for review by special agreement

Copying: This journal has been registered with the Copyright Clearance Center (CCC), as indicated by the code appearing on the first page of each article.
For readers in the US, this code signals consent for copying of articles for personal or internal use, or for the personal or internal use of specific clients, provided that the stated fee is paid per copy directly to
Copyright Clearance Center Inc.
222 Rosewood Drive
Danvers, MA 01923 (USA)
A copy of the first page of the article must accompany payment. Consent does not extend to copying for general distribution, for promotion, for creating new works, or for resale. In these cases, specific written permission must be obtained from the copyright owner,
S. Karger AG,
P.O. Box, CH–4009 Basel (Switzerland).

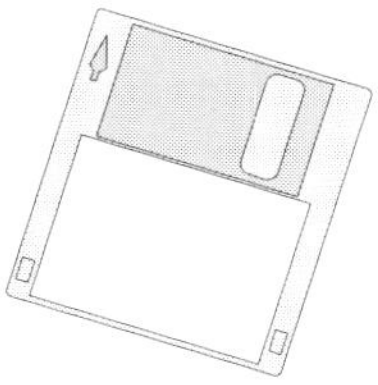

Disk Submission

A **comprehensive version** of these guidelines for the **submission of manuscripts and illustrations on disk** can be accessed online under **www.karger.com/journals/disksub.htm** or requested as a leaflet from the editorial department.

Please follow the general rules on style and arrangement in the **"Guidelines for Authors"** of the journal. Submit a **double-spaced printout** of your manuscript matching the file on disk exactly.

Technical Information

Store only data pertinent to this manuscript. Include your fonts (screen and printer fonts for Macintosh). For a **text only** manuscript, use a 3.5 inch disk. For **text and illustrations,** use 3.5 or 5.25 Magneto Optical Disc; CD-ROM (DOS or hybrid); iomage Zip/DOS (100 MB), or 44 MB, 88 MB or 200 MB SyQuest. Compress extensive data using ZIP format.

Data Description

Label your disk with the **title of the journal or book** for which it is submitted; a **short version** of the paper's title; your **name,** postal and e-mail address, fax and phone number; **hard and software** used, including the version; and the **complete list of the file names.** File names consist of eight characters before the dot identifying the file and three characters after the dot identifying the application.

Text and Format

The **preferred word-processing package is MS-Word.** Other commonly used PC text programs and ASCII formats are accepted.
Update your data when you revise subsequent to the reviewer's or editor's decision and mark revisions clearly. Manuscripts accepted for publication are subject to **copy editing:** changes and/or questions will be marked in the manuscript, which will be returned to you with your disk and the galley proofs for checking.
Enter your text continuously flush left. Do not use any layout functions. Do not split words at the end of a line. **Do not use indentations.** Use a blank line before and a hard return at the end of paragraphs.
Arrange headings flush left. Insert only **one space after punctuation marks.** Insert Greek letters, mathematical symbols etc. with your word-processing program. Use **boldface and italics** as well as sub- and superscript where appropriate.
Tables are part of the text and should be placed at the end of the text file. Separate the individual parts of a table by lines. Use the tabulator instead of spaces. Format operation data on one line in the same column. **Legends to illustrations are part of the text** and should also be listed at the end of the text file.

Illustrations

Store illustrations as separate files: do not embed them in your text. Export **line drawings/vector graphics** as TIF, EPS or WMF format. Use Photoshop for processing and retouching **scanned halftone images.** Save the original scan and the processed version. Export **black and white or color images** as TIF or EPS format in their anticipated size in print.
For detailed information on how to submit illustration data on disk please consult the leaflet or **www.karger.com/journals/disksub.htm.**

© 1999 S. Karger AG, Basel

The Journal Home Page is available at:
www.karger.com/journals/orl

KI 98 DISK

50. Tagung der Oto-Rhino-Laryngologischen Gesellschaft zu München e.V.

München, Deutschland, 4.–5. Dezember 1999

Thema

Hals-Nasen-Ohren-Heilkunde,
heute und morgen

Präsidenten

Professor Dr. E. Kastenbauer
Professor Dr. W. Arnold

Organisation

Professor Dr. G. Grevers

Sekretariat

Frau Marlies Herzog
HNO-Klink im Klinikum Grosshadern
Marchioninistr. 15
D–81377 München

Tel.: +49 89 70 95 38 67
Fax: +49 89 70 95 88 25
E-Mail: mherzog@hno.med.uni-muenchen.de

F 99403

Karger Journals in **ORL**

***O**utstanding coverage*
***R**ewarding reading*
***L**eading contributions - in our journal program*

Audiology & Neuro-Otology

ORL

Oto-Rhino-Laryngologia Nova

Folia Phoniatrica et Logopaedica

Phonetica

KARGER

Please ask for free sample copies

KI99433g

ORL

Cochlear Mechanics

Guest Editor
Frank Böhnke, Munich, Germany

91 figures, 3 in color, 4 tables, 1999

KARGER

Basel · Freiburg · Paris · London · New York ·
New Delhi · Bangkok · Singapore · Tokyo · Sydney

S. Karger
Medical and Scientific Publishers
Basel · Freiburg · Paris · London
New York · New Delhi · Bangkok
Singapore · Tokyo · Sydney

Drug Dosage
The authors and the publisher have exerted every effort to ensure that drug selection and dosage set forth in this text are in accord with current recommendations and practice at the time of publication. However, in view of ongoing research, changes in government regulations, and the constant flow of information relating to drug therapy and drug reactions, the reader is urged to check the package insert for each drug for any change in indications and dosage and for added warnings and precautions. This is particularly important when the recommended agent is a new and/or infrequently employed drug.

All rights reserved.
No part of this publication may be translated into other languages, reproduced or utilized in any form or by any means, electronic or mechanical, including photocopying, recording, microcopying, or by any information storage and retrieval system, without permission in writing from the publisher or, in the case of photocopying, direct payment of a specified fee to the Copyright Clearance Center (see 'General Information').

© Copyright 1999 by S. Karger AG,
P.O. Box, CH–4009 Basel (Switzerland)
Printed in Switzerland on acid-free paper by
Reinhardt Druck, Basel
ISBN 3–8055–6988–2

KARGER

Fax+ 41 61 306 12 34
E-Mail karger@karger.ch
www.karger.com

Vol. 61, No. 5, 1999

ORL

Contents

KARGER

Fax+ 41 61 306 12 34
E-Mail karger@karger.ch
www.karger.com

© 1999 S. Karger AG, Basel

Access to full text and tables of contents, including tentative ones for forthcoming issues:
www.karger.com/journals/orl/orl_bk.htm

ORL

ORL 1999;61:237

Introduction

It is our pleasure to present nine unique articles on the topic of 'Cochlear Mechanics'. Today it is clear that cochlear mechanics are influenced by electric signals on afferent and efferent nerve endings at the cells of the organ of Corti. Therefore, limiting the processes in the cochlea to mechanical aspects must be conceptually wrong. On the other hand, if we recognize that many workers of diverse disciplines in otology use the facts from cochlear mechanics for the interpretation of their results, we think it is more than reasonable to dedicate a complete issue of this journal to this topic.

Owing to the strong interdisciplinarity of the articles it is not only interesting for ENT clinicians but also for biophysicists, biomechanical engineers, audio engineers, radiologists, electrophysiologists, applied mathematicians and perhaps others too.

Ch.R. Steele gives a review on cochlear modeling and indicates that several traveling waves are present in the cochlea and that the pressures in the inner fluid regions of the organ of Corti can be large. Two articles show the close connection between otoacoustic emissions and cochlear mechanics (H. Wada, T. Nakajima and K. Ohyama; M. Ganz and M. Berg). An important approach for future cochlear modeling is shown by the work of U. Vogel who is able to produce geometrical data for the input of three-dimensional finite element models by microtomographic imaging. The careful reader of the inner ear literature has mentioned a returning interest in cochlear fluid mechanics, and I thank E.-J. Haberland and H.J. Neumann for letting us have the experimental results which were difficult to obtain. A remarkable article by A. Spector tries to prove a connection between outer hair cell mechanics and the complex phenomenon tinnitus and is in addition a 'delicacy' for stress engineers who usually calculate the mechanics of rockets, airplanes or cars. Following the steps of former reseachers who modeled the mechanics of the cochlea by electrical network components (e.g. Peterson and Bogart, Oetinger and Hauser, Zwicker, DeBoer, Allen), F. Baumgarte uses the concept of wave-digital filters and draws conclusions regarding psychoacoustics which are relevant for example for the transmission of music over the World Wide Web.

In my opinion, a milestone in understanding cochlear mechanics is set by the claim that otoacoustic emissions are generated by the superposition of signals produced by vulnerable physiological processes and reflection components in the cochlea [Evoked otoacoustic emissions arise by two fundamentally different mechanisms: A taxonomy for mammalian OAEs; Shera and Guinan Jr: J Acoust Soc Am, Feb 1999]. With this in mind it is a natural consequence to develop three-dimensional mechanical models of the cochlea including fluid-structure couplings, and the micromechanical truss built by the cells of the cochlear partition including the stereocilia and the tectorial membrane.

Of course an article on the mechanics of the sterocilia bundle of hair cells is missing. Although there are already promising studies which cover it, I hope this topic is picked up further in the future and brought in the context of macromechanical cochlear models.

Though I think we have made remarkable progress in analyzing cochlear mechanics, the following still seems to be true: 'Cochlear technology itself is a step or two ahead of us still' [David Kemp, Feb. 1999].

Munich, May 1999

Frank Böhnke

KARGER

Fax + 41 61 306 12 34
E-Mail karger@karger.ch
www.karger.com

© 1999 S. Karger AG, Basel

Accessible online at:
http://BioMedNet.com/karger

ORL

ORL 1999;61:238–251

Toward Three-Dimensional Analysis of Cochlear Structure

Charles R. Steele

Division of Mechanics and Computation, Department of Mechanical Engineering, Stanford University, Stanford, Calif., USA

Key Words

Model · Cochlea · Sulcus · Elastic · Viscous · WKB · Stiffness · Waves

Abstract

Recent results from a three-dimensional model of the cochlea are summarized. The features include physically realistic values of basilar membrane stiffness, mass, and fluid viscosity. The simple 'feed-forward' principle for the active process yields results in qualitative agreement with recent mesurements in the cochlea. The limitation is a simplified representation of the organ of Corti, with two degrees of freedom representing the motion of the pectinate and arcuate zones of the basilar membrane. However, the inner sulcus fluid flow is included. The new feature presented in this paper is an approach to treat all the structural detail of the organ of Corti, with the sole input to the calculation in a form easily understood by anyone familiar with the cochlea. Specific results are shown for the Pakistani water buffalo, since a fairly complete anatomical description of this cochlea is available. The static stiffness from the calculation, based on only the anatomy and known values for the protein elastic moduli, are in remarkable agreement with recent measurements in the gerbil cochlea. Only preliminary results for the dynamic response with inviscid fluid are reported. Of interest, however, are the propagation modes related to significant fluid displacement and pressure in the different compartments of the organ of Corti.

Introduction

The cochlea is an elaborate organ with many components, each of which is crafted for a significant purpose and for significant interaction with each other (fig. 1). The advance in computing power opens the possibility of including more of the components into a mathematical model. With such computations, speculation can be reduced and interpretation of experiments improved. Direct numerical treatment by a finite difference mesh of the entire cochlea remains a formidable challenge for the newest computers. For reasonable details of the full-length cochlea, organ of Corti, and the viscous fluid, the solution of a matrix with dimensions around 50 million is required, just to calculate the linear response to a single frequency. Nevertheless, versions of the direct numerical approach are under development in several laboratories. The first extensive effort to use the finite element method to model the details of the cochlea and the organ of Corti, with a physical basis for all parameters, is by Raftenberg [20]. Kolston and Ashmore [14] have generated more

KARGER

Fax + 41 61 306 12 34
E-Mail karger@karger.ch
www.karger.com

© 1999 S. Karger AG, Basel
0301–1569/99/0615–0238$17.50/0

Accessible online at:
http://BioMedNet.com/karger

Charles R. Steele
Division of Mechanics and Computation, Department of Mechanical Engineering
Durand Building, Room 262, Stanford University
Stanford, CA 94305 (USA)
E-Mail chasst@leland.stanford.edu

Fig. 1. Fast4 calculation for the deformation of the cochlear partition due to pressure on the basilar membrane (BM). Outer hair cell (OHC) stereocilia are sheared by the motion of the pillars of Corti and reticular lamina relative to the tectorial membrane (TM). The basilar membrane is supported on the left by the bony shelf and on the right by the spiral ligament. The inner hair cells (IHC) are the primary receptors, each with about 20 afferent synapses. The inner sulcus (IC) is a fluid region in contact with the cilia of the inner hair cells. Scala tympani (ST) is the fluid region on the lower side, while scala media is above the organ. For the calculation without the Reissner's membrane, scala media and scala vestibuli (SV) are the same fluid.

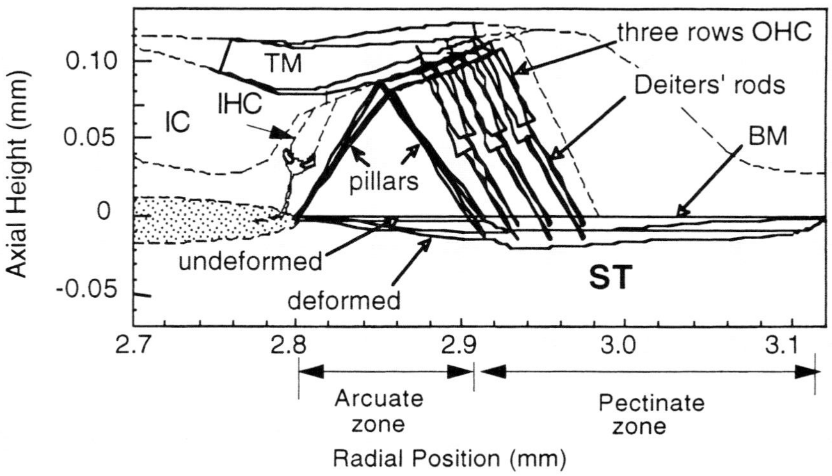

details of the response with a finite element code, that includes three-dimensional details of the organ of Corti and the fluid. However, they cannot yet include curvature of the cochlea, the elements of the organ of Corti must be rectangular, and the viscosity of the fluid is not included. The elements representing the fluid and the elastic structures are somewhat unorthodox, and no verification calculations are reported. Still, the computing time requirement is such that massive parallel computing would be required for the response at a fixed point in the cochlea for a frequency sweep, or for consideration of an iterative process for treating nonlinearities. Böhnke et al. [3] use the commercial code ANSYS to develop the most accurate model of the organ of Corti, including the spatial geometry of the discrete hair cells and Dieter's rods and processes. However, computer memory limitations restrict them to a fairly small length of the cochlea and fluid is not included. Zhang et al. [36] presented beautiful results for the resonance of the cochlear cross section. However, they also do not include the fluid; consequently, the resonant frequency computed is rather high. What they simulate confirms Békésy's observation [1] that the drained cochlea has no significant partition resonance in the auditory range. A three-dimensional solution for inviscid fluid using the finite element program SEPRAN is by van Hengel [12] who includes a plan to extent this to include details of the organ of Corti. Thus, there is substantial interest in developing computation methods for the full three-dimensional details of the cochlea.

In contrast to a direct numerical solution, a combination of numerical and perturbation methods is appealing. The typical mammalian cochlea has cross-sectional geometry that varies with the distance from the stapes. However, this variation is 'slow', i.e., the wavelength of the actual response is small in comparison with the distance over which the properties vary significantly. For such systems, the application of the method, referred to as 'LG', 'WKB', 'phase-integral' or 'physical optics', provides an efficient procedure for capturing the significant behavior. The pioneering effort in this directon is by Ranke [21], as discussed by Siebert [25], and extended to the two-dimensional cochlear model by Steele [26]. This work shows that the waves in the cochlea near the maximum are 'short wave' and dispersive. Direct confirmation of the three-dimensional fluid behavior is from the in vivo pressure measurements by Olson [18], which are similar to the three-dimensional calculations by Taber and Steele [34].

It is important to validate computational results with direct comparison with experimental physical models. The three-dimensional calculation [33] produced results in reasonable agreement with measurements in the experimental Model K by Helle [11]. Model K was without organ of Corti and 6 times life-sized. Helle measured all fluid and basilar membrane viscoelastic properties, so there were no free parameters for 'adjusting' results. The recent experimental model by Zhou et al. [37] is valuable since it is the first life-sized physical experimental model and therefore requires no scaling. However, a viscosity of the fluid 28 times that of saline was used for optical purposes, and the exact thickness of the basilar membrane is not given. Our computations for this case with a reasonable taper in the basilar membrane thickness are in rea-

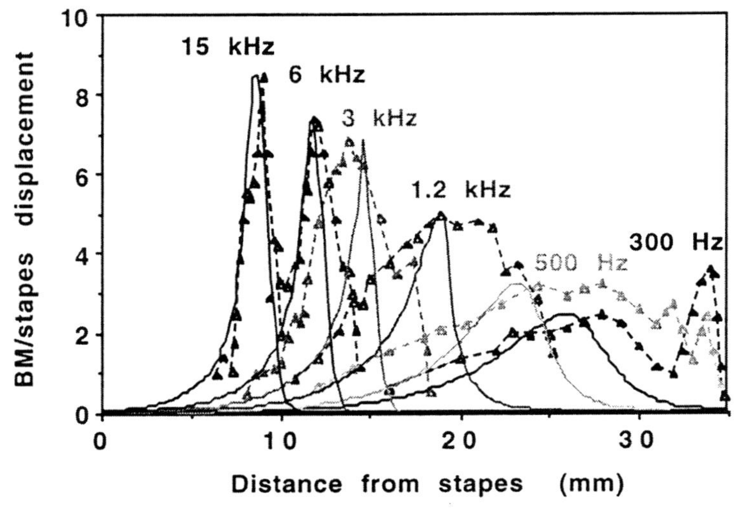

Fig. 2. Comparison of 3-D model calculations (solid curves) with experimental results of Zhou et a. [37] (dashed curves) for the amplitude envelopes for different frequencies. This is a life-size model, but with an isotropic BM and fluid viscosity 28 times that of water. The agreement is reasonable, except for the lower frequencies.

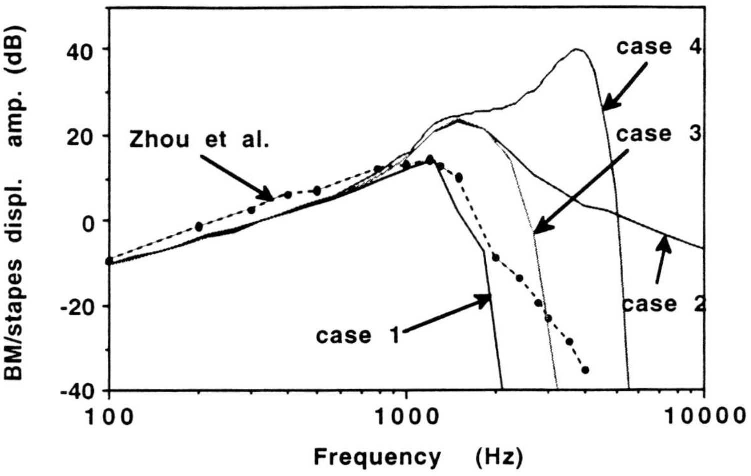

Fig. 3. Comparison of 3-D model calculations with experimental results of Zhou et al. [37] for amplitude at the place $\chi = 19$ mm as a function of frequency. The scales are logarithmic (20 dB is a factor of 10 in amplitude). Case 1 shows a direct comparison with the physical parameters of the experiment, with isotropic BM and viscosity 28 times that of water. Case 2 is computed for the viscosity reduced to that of water. Case 3 is computed for the BM made of transverse fibers. Case 4 shows the effect of active OHC feed-forward, with the pressure ain $\alpha = 0.21$ and feed-forward distance $\Delta\chi = 25$ µm. Thus lower viscosity, BM orthotropy and active feed-forward all contribute to higher amplitude and increased localization of the response.

sonable agreement, as shown in figures 2 and 3 from Steele et al., [30]. So the approach seems to yield good numerical results at low computational cost. Typically, the response of the cochlear model without organ of Corti for one frequency requires a few seconds of computation.

It appears that the inclination of the outer hair cells in the longitudinal direction is important for the active process. A simple 'feed-forward' relation for an active model without organ of Corti is proposed by Steele et al. [28], which has been also used by Geisler and Sang [9].

Including the Organ of Corti

It is clear that the WKB method is efficient for computation and provides excellent results for the simple cochlear model without the organ of Corti. This paper reports the progress in extending the approach to include more details of the organ of Corti. From measurements by Khanna et al. [13] and by Gummer et al. [10], the independent resonance of the tectorial membrane must play an important role. We seek the capability of including all such detail.

Several more elaborate multichamber models of the cochlea have been studied. Boulet [4] considered the larger experimental models containing an 'organ of Corti' (models G1 and G2, 30 times life-size [11] with the WKB method. However, the results were not satisfactory, in that substantial discrepancies between measurement and computational results existed. Multichamber models have also been considered with a modification of WKB by Fuhrmann et al. [8] and Chadwick and Dimitriades [6]. Generally, each additional chamber provides an additional mode of wave propagation.

A first step is to include the fluid in the inner sulcus shown in figure 1. Since the fluid pressure of this region acts directly on the inner hair cells, one can argue that the purpose of the entire organ of Corti is to develop the inner sulcus pressure. The inner sulcus is considered by de Boer [2] and Steele and Lim [32]. The feed-forward active process can be expressed for this model as well.

As indicated by the measurements of Ruggero et al. [23] shown in figure 4, the cochlear response is dependent on the level of acoustic stimulation. Adding the active feed-forward [28, 32] produces the results shown in figure 5. This is a linear computation, but the amplitude of the feed-forward gain is changed. A substantial increase of the amplitude of response is the consequence of a small value of the feed-forward gain. The measured phase in the cochlea is in figure 6 and the calculated values in figure 7. The qualitative features of the measurement and computation are similar. Particularly, the phase is insensitive to the amplitude of stimulus, and in the calculation is insensitive to the magnitude of the feed-forward gain. A nonlinear computation has been carried out, in which the feed-forward gain saturates with amplitude of input. The results are similar to those in figures 5 and 7. So with completely reasonable physical parameters, the mathematical computation yields reasonable results. The conclusion expressed in the title by Naidu and Mountain [17] is true for one-dimensional cochlear models, but not for realistic three-dimensional models.

What does not agree with the cochlear measurements is the shift of the characteristic frequency (CF) from the passive to the active. The calculation show about a one octave shift while the measurements typically show a one-half octave shift. The feed-forward gain in this calculation is, however, constant. The detailed behavior of the hair cell is not included. We expect that the electrical behavior of the cell [19] and the electromechanical interaction will have a substantial effect in reducing the gain for high frequencies, which should shift the computed peak to a lower frequency. A point worth noting is that the long wave-

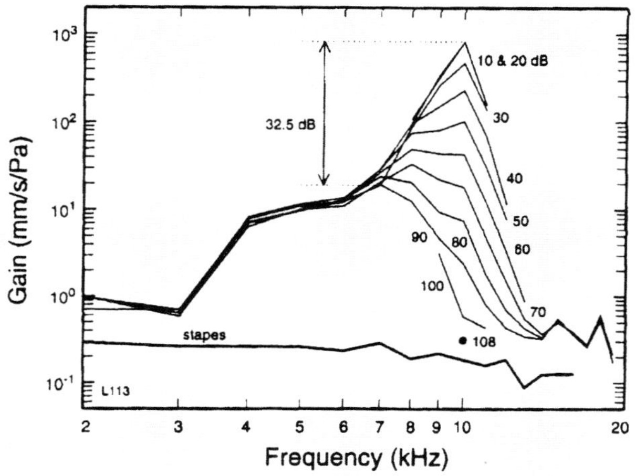

Fig. 4. Response to tones of chinchilla cochlea at point 3.5 mm from round window, from Ruggero et al. [23]. The gain is the amplitude of basilar-membrane velocity divided by the stimulus pressure (animal L113).

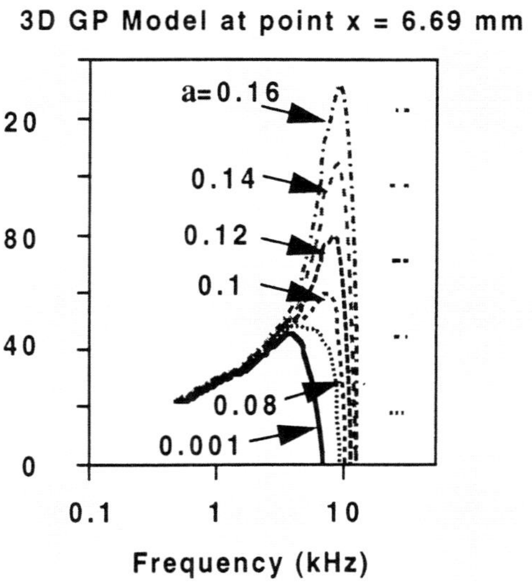

Fig. 5. Response of 3-D model for guinea pig cochlea with different values for the feed-forward gain. with modest feed-forward amplitude α, an 80-dB increase of the BM amplitude is achieved. From Steele and Lim [32].

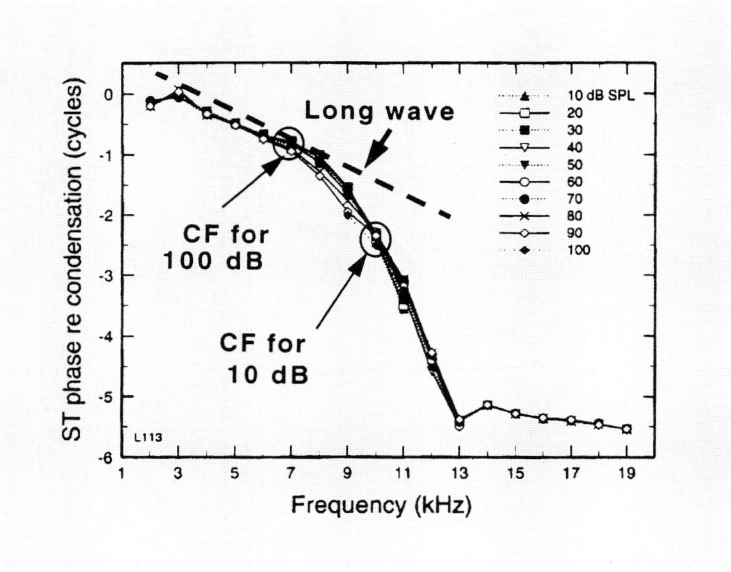

Fig. 6. Phase associated with the amplitude in figure 4, from Ruggero et al. [23] (animal L113). The phase is remarkably insensitive to the stimulus amplitude. We have added the circles that show the points of maximum displacement for different values of stimulus and the dashed line to indicate the long wavelength portion of the response.

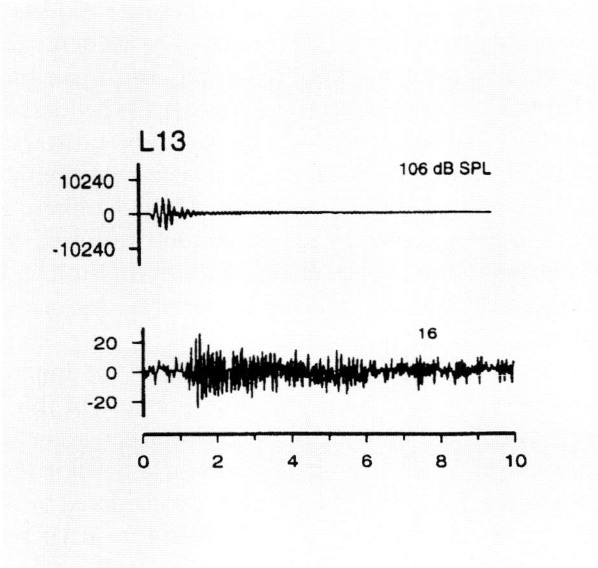

Fig. 8. Basilar membrane response to condensationclicks at high stimulus level of 106 dB and low level of 16 dB. From Recio et al. [22]. Note the more extensive ringing for the low level, at which the active process is significant.

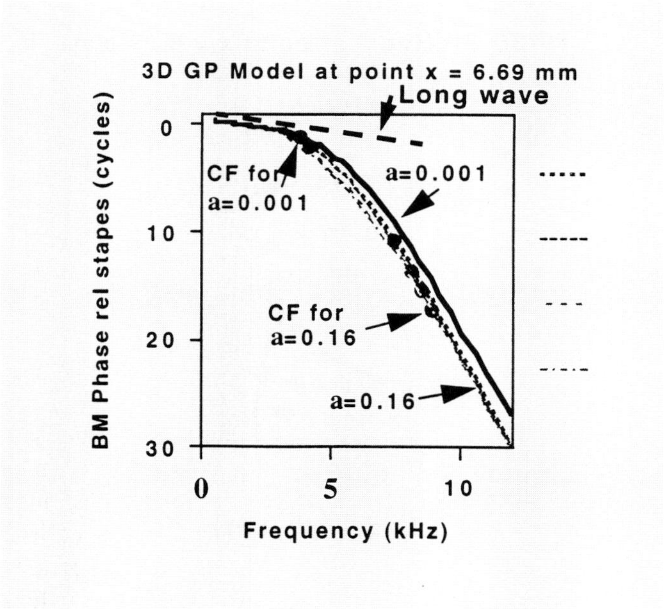

Fig. 7. Phase associated with the amplitude in figure 5. The phase is remarkably insensitive to the gain. The dots show the points of maximum displacement for different values of the feed-forward gain. From Steele and Lim [32].

length behavior is characterized by a linear relation between phase and frequency. The experiments figure 6 normally show a deviation from linear as CF is approached. This is further evidence that the fluid motion is short wavelength in the vicinity of CF.

Transient response has also been calculated. In figure 8 are measurements from Recio et al. [22] which show prolonged ringing for low amplitude of stimulus. The calculated response [15] to a sharp click are in figure 9 which also show prolonged ringing when the feed-forward gain is on.

Therefore, much can be obtained from the simplified models without the organ of Corti and the active behavior of the outer hair cells represented by a feed-forward pressure gain. Adding the inner sulcus in a rough approximate manner is better. Better yet would be the complete calculation of the elements of the organ of Corti exactly as they are.

A major effort of the past years has been on the computer program 'Fast4', discussed by Steele and Shad [29]. This is a program for the computation of the dynamic response of complex shell structures. Perturbation and numerical methods are combined to obtain orders of

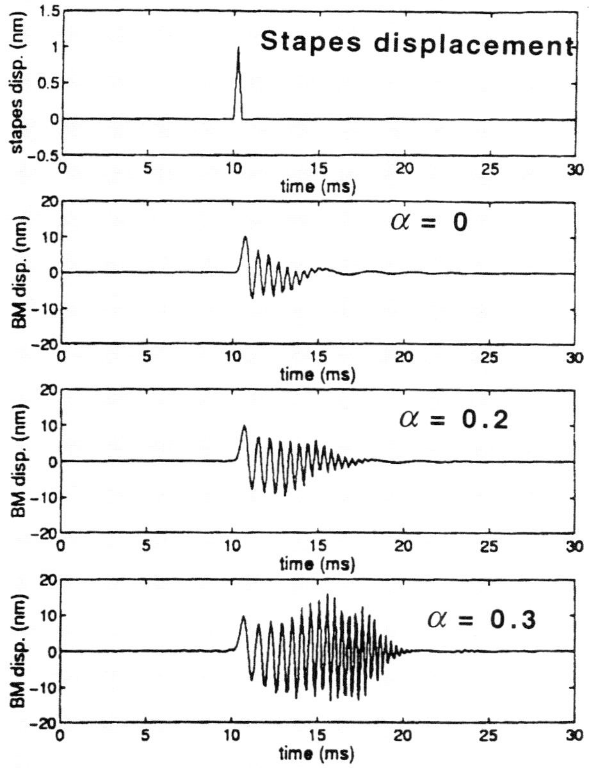

Fig. 9. Model response to a sharp click input to the stapes, shown in the upper plot. The lower plots show the response on the basilar membrane for the passive case $\alpha = 0$, and active feed-forward cases of $\alpha = 0.2$ and $\alpha = 0.3$. The feed-forward causes additional ringing. From Lim and Steele [15].

reduction in both user preparation time and computation time, in comparison with commercial finite element programs. With Fast4 virtually all the structural detail of the actual cross section of the cochlea can be computed. Some preliminary examples of the application to the hearing organ of lizards birds, and the mustached bat are in Steele [31]. In figure 1 is an example of the deformation of the guinea pig cochlear cross section with static mechanical loading, consisting of vacuum in the lower fluid region. each structure is modelled as on orthotropic shell of revolution. The computational time for one frequency of excitation of such a structure is now reduced to about 15 s (Mac G3 laptop, 300 MHz).

Water Buffalo Cochlea

To compute the details of the organ of Corti, the dimensions of the individual components are needed. It appears, however, that the most complete measurement of the dimensions as a function of the distance along the cochlea is provided by Tiedemann [35] for the Pakistani water buffalo *(Anoa bubalis)*. The entries in table 1 are mainly taken from his tabulated values at the distances from the stapes of 10, 19, 25, 30, 33 and 36 mm. The values at the stapes STdis = 0 are obtained by extrapolation. However, Tiedemann did not provide all the necessary dimensions, so some values are estimated. The elastic properties for the elements are taken simply as 1 GPa for the elements consisting of elastin, collagen, and microtubules. (From point load measurements in the guinea pig, Miller [16] estimated the modulus of basilar membrane fibers to be 1.9 GPa.) The volume fraction of 0.1 from the fibers for the basilar membrane is from Cabezudo [5] and a value for the volume fraction of the protein fibers in the tectorial membrane taken as 0.001. Tiedemann's micrographs indicate considerable distortion, so that actual values could be quite different, but we presume that the variation along the cochlea will be correct. Reissner's membrane and the details of the primary spiral osseous lamina should also be included. Table 1 indicates, however, the information needed for a detailed computation. It is desirable to have such dimensions for human and the usual laboratory animals.

Analysis

The objective is to have a simple input that can be used for any cochlea and reasonable computation time for the response. The first is accomplished by having table 1 provide the only input for the computation. With a little more explanation of the notation, these quantities are readily understood by anyone with knowledge of the cochlea. To achieve a reasonable computation time, the approximation is made that (1) all the inertia and damping is in the fluid and (2) that the elastic response of the cross section is independent of the wavelength, which corresponds to negligible elastic coupling in the longitudinal direction. Thus the elastic behavior of each of the six cross sections needs to be computed only once. The compliance values are then interpolated (on a logarithmic scale) to obtain values for a fine mesh along the cochlea. The three-dimensional fluid response for each subregion is a faster calculation. Thus the procedure is the following.

Table 1. Model for Pakistani water buffalo (from Tiedemann [35])

		Distance from stapes (STdis)						
		0	10	19	25	30	33	36
Basilar membrane	BMwidthAZ	0.030	0.050	0.065	0.073	0.083	0.090	0.105
	BMthickAZ	0.0056	0.0049	0.004	0.0033	0.0027	0.0024	0.002
	BMwidthPZ	0.06	0.12	0.17	0.22	0.25	0.27	0.30
	BMthickPZ	0.015	0.0100	0.008	0.0066	0.0052	0.0048	0.004
	BMvolFract	0.1	0.1	0.1	0.1	0.1	0.1	0.1
	BMyD1	0.005	0.01	0.013	0.018	0.02	0.021	0.025
	BMyD2	0.01	0.02	0.026	0.036	0.04	0.042	0.050
	BMyD3	0.015	0.03	0.039	0.054	0.06	0.063	0.075
	BMyHC	0.02	0.04	0.054	0.071	0.081	0.09	0.10
	BMemod	0.1×10^{10}	0.1×10^{10}	0.1×10^{10}	0.1×10^{10}	0.1×10^{10}	0.1×10^{10}	0.1×10^{10}
Pillars	Py	0.0150	0.0302	0.0492	0.0561	0.0615	0.065	0.0713
	Pz	0.0195	0.0195	0.0196	0.0286	0.0334	0.0308	0.0231
	Pdia	0.0027	0.0027	0.0028	0.0029	0.0031	0.003	0.0029
	Pemod	0.1×10^{10}	0.1×10^{10}	0.1×10^{10}	0.1×10^{10}	0.1×10^{10}	0.1×10^{10}	0.1×10^{10}
Cross section	Rad0	3.7	3.4	3.06	2.72	2.38	2.04	1.7
	SVheight	1.0	1.0	1.0	1.0	1.0	1.0	1.0
	SVheight	1.0	1.0	1.0	1.0	1.0	1.0	1.0
	STheight	1.0	1.0	1.0	1.0	1.0	1.0	1.0
	STwidth	1.0	1.0	1.0	1.0	1.0	1.0	1.0
Reticular lamina	RTdisOCH1	0.008	0.015	0.027	0.032	0.035	0.037	0.038
	RTdisOHC2	0.014	0.025	0.037	0.042	0.045	0.047	0.048
	RTdisOHC3	0.023	0.035	0.047	0.052	0.055	0.057	0.058
	RTdisHen	0.030	0.040	0.060	0.075	0.085	0.090	0.100
	RTthick	0.001	0.001	0.001	0.001	0.001	0.001	0.001
	RTangle	53.0	43.0	37.3	24.3	17.3	12.5	6.1
	RTemod	0.1×10^{10}	0.1×10^{10}	0.1×10^{10}	0.1×10^{10}	0.1×10^{10}	0.1×10^{10}	0.1×10^{10}
Outer hair cells	OHCdia	0.0069	0.0072	0.0075	0.0077	0.0072	0.008	0.008
	OHClength	0.022	0.025	0.028	0.032	0.036	0.038	0.040
	OHCwallThick	0.1×10^{-5}	0.1×10^{-5}	0.1×10^{-5}	0.1×10^{-5}	0.1×10^{-5}	0.1×10^{-5}	0.1×10^{-5}
	OHCemod	0.1×10^{10}	0.1×10^{10}	0.1×10^{10}	0.1×10^{10}	0.1×10^{10}	0.1×10^{10}	0.1×10^{10}
Cilia	CLength	0.0031	0.0029	0.0022	0.0021	0.002	0.0019	0.0018
	CDia	0.00030	0.00028	0.00028	0.00021	0.00019	0.00019	0.00018
	CNumber	125	125	125	125	125	125	125
	CDiaBase	0.00009	0.00009	0.00009	0.00007	0.00006	0.00006	0.000006
	CHeightBase	0.00028	0.00028	0.00028	0.00021	0.00019	0.00019	0.00018
	Cemod	0.1×10^{10}	0.1×10^{10}	0.1×10^{10}	0.1×10^{10}	0.1×10^{10}	0.1×10^{10}	0.1×10^{10}
Dieter cells	DCdia	0.0027	0.0027	0.0028	0.0029	0.0031	0.003	0.0029
	DCemod	0.1×10^{10}	0.1×10^{10}	0.1×10^{10}	0.1×10^{10}	0.1×10^{10}	0.1×10^{10}	0.1×10^{10}
Tectorial membrane (TM)	TMy0	–0.06	–0.08	–0.16	–0.21	–0.25	–0.28	–0.3
	TMz0	0.039	0.039	0.039	0.0572	0.0668	0.0616	0.0462
	TMthick0	0.026	0.026	0.020	0.015	0.012	0.011	0.010
	TMthickP	0.008	0.008	0.006	0.0052	0.0036	0.0033	0.003
	TMthickOHC1	0.008	0.008	0.006	0.0052	0.0036	0.0033	0.003
	TMthickOHC2	0.008	0.008	0.006	0.0052	0.0036	0.0033	0.003
	TMthickOCH3	0.008	0.008	0.006	0.0052	0.0033	0.0033	0.003
	TMthickHen	0.008	0.008	0.006	0.0052	0.0036	0.0033	0.003
	TMvolFract	0.001	0.001	0.001	0.001	0.001	0.001	0.001
	TMemod	0.1×10^{10}	0.1×10^{10}	0.1×10^{10}	0.1×10^{10}	0.1×10^{10}	0.1×10^{10}	0.1×10^{10}
Hensen cells	HCthick0	0.0027	0.0027	0.0028	0.0029	0.0031	0.003	0.0029
	HCthick1	0.0027	0.0027	0.0028	0.0029	0.0031	0.003	0.0029
	HCemod	0.1×10^{4}	0.1×10^{4}	0.1×10^{4}	0.1×10^{4}	0.1×10^{4}	0.1×10^{4}	0.1×10^{4}

Values at STdis = 0 are extrapolated.
Values of cochlear parameters: all lengths in mm, Young's modulus (emod) in Pa.

Process data: An interface program has been written that reads the file consisting of table 1 and automatically generates the input data files for Fast4.

Elastic computation: The elastic response of each section is computed automatically with the execution of Gast4. The results are placed in the form of a flexibility matrix F:

$$V = F \cdot P \tag{1}$$

where P is a vector of pressures acting on each structural element of the cross section, currently 22 in number, while V is the vector of corresponding area displacements. (Actually, cylindrical coordinates are used, so V is the integral of the displacement multiplied by the radius from the axis of the cochlea.) The maxtrix F should be symmetric and with positive diagonal terms.

Reduction to fluid regions: The fluid regions are identified. For this preliminary effort, we consider six fluid regions: (1) SV: scala vestibuli – scala media; (2) ST: scala tympani; (3) IS: inner sulcus; (4) T: tunnel region formed by the pillars and the arcuate zone of the basilar membrane; (5) OHC: outer hair cell region, bounded by the outer pillar, the recticular lamina, the Hensen cells, and the pectinate zone of the basilar membrane, and (6) STML: fluid layer between the tectorial membrane and the recticular lamina. At this time, the leaking from one region to the other, i.e., between regions (4) and (5) through the outer pillars, is not taken into consideration. Indeed it will be better to have regions (5) and (6) subdivided into four regions, and the leaking around the hair cells and cilia included. For the fluid flow, the total area displacement of each region is important. This can be obtained from the displacements of the 22 structural elements in equation 1 by a reduction matrix R:

$$V_R = R \cdot V \tag{2}$$

where V_R is the vector of area displacements of the six fluid regions. Thus the dimensional size of the reduction matrix is 6×22. Using this in equation 1 gives a reduced flexibility matrix F_R:

$$V_R = F_R \cdot P_R \tag{3}$$

where the reduced matrix is computed from:

$$F_R = R \cdot F \cdot R^T \tag{4}$$

and P_R is a reduced vector of pressures:

$$P = R^T \cdot P_R \tag{5}$$

The elements of P_R give the net effective pressure acting on the wall, while the elements of V_R give the net area displacement of the walls of each fluid region. Thus, the fluid motion in the duct can be calculated in terms of the elements of P_R and V_R. So the problem begins with the solution for the continuous elastic structure, e.g. infinite degrees of freedom, and is reduced to a small system (eq. 3), without losing the essential physics of the behavior.

Fluid solution: The local behavior of each fluid region can be computed. The simplest approximation is to treat each region as an equivalent rectangle and use the three-dimensional calculation in Taber and Steele [33] or the improved version in Steele and Lim [32]. For the local solution, we consider all quantities to vary as:

$$\begin{bmatrix} P_R \\ V_R \end{bmatrix} \leftarrow \begin{bmatrix} P_R \\ V_R \end{bmatrix} \exp\left(\omega t - \int_0^x n dx\right) \tag{6}$$

where ω is the frequency and n is the wave number. With this, the relation between the pressure and area displacement is obtained in the form:

$$P_R = \rho\omega^2 H \cdot V_R \tag{7}$$

where ρ is the density of the fluid, ω is the frequency, and H is a matrix. Presently, H has only diagonal terms, but leaking between fluid regions will add coupling terms. The elements of H depend on the wave number and the fluid viscosity and frequency. For inviscid fluid there is no dependence on frequency. For example, the one- and two-dimensional approximations for the solution for a inviscid fluid region are:

$$H = \begin{cases} \dfrac{1}{n^2 bh} & \text{for 1-D} \\ \dfrac{1}{nb \tanh nh} & \text{for 2-D} \end{cases} \tag{8}$$

in which b is the width of the region, and h is the height above the moving surface. The three-dimensional solution with fluid viscosity involves summing Fourier series across the width of the region.

Fluid-elastic interaction. The local wave propagation properties are determined from the elasticity (eq. 3) and the fluid (eq. 7), which may be written together as:

$$\begin{bmatrix} -I & \rho\omega^2 H \\ F_R & -I \end{bmatrix} \cdot \begin{bmatrix} P_R \\ V_R \end{bmatrix} = \begin{bmatrix} 0 \\ 0 \end{bmatrix} \tag{9}$$

In general, an iterative procedure in the complex plane must be used to find the wave number for a given frequency for which a solution of this system can be found. The search is assisted however, by considering first the inviscid fluid. The H is independent of frequency and equation 9 reduces to the standard eigenvalue problem:

$$\left[F_R \cdot H - \frac{1}{\rho\omega^2} I\right] \cdot V_R = 0 \tag{10}$$

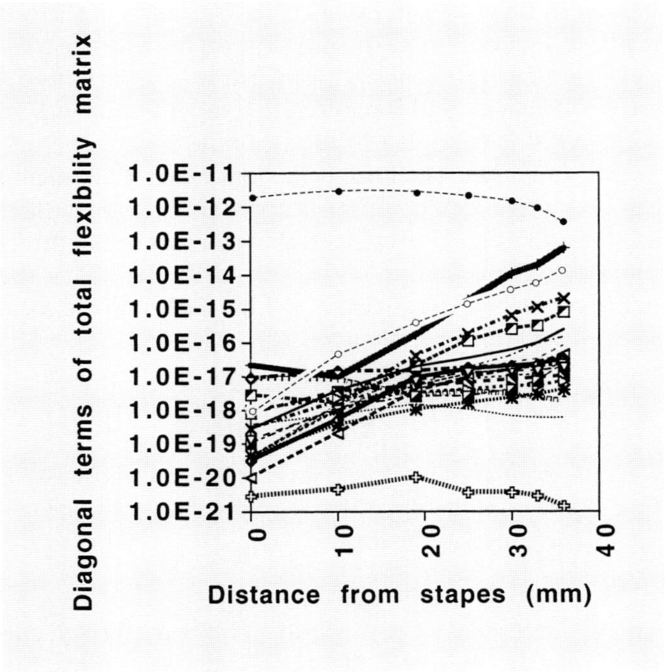

Fig. 10. The diagonal terms of the total flexibility matrix computed by Fast4 for the buffalo cochlea from the entries in table 1. Note that the slopes the individual flexibility terms are not at all the same.

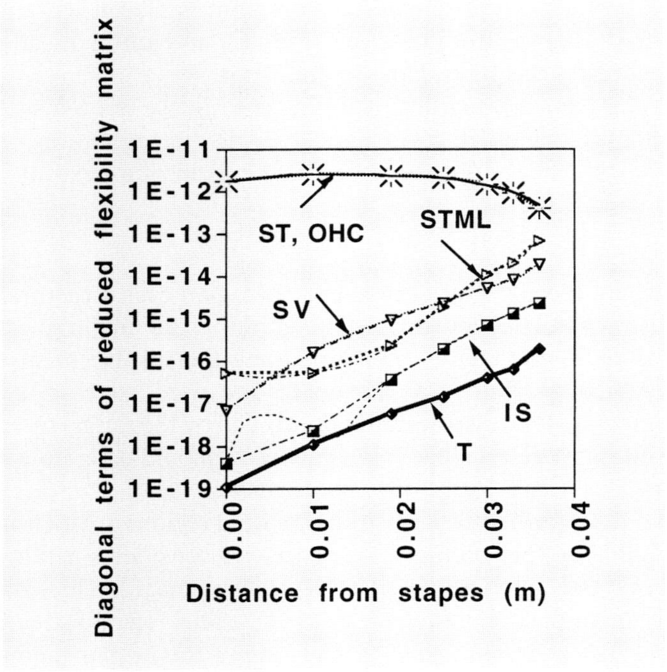

Fig. 11. The diagonal terms of the reduced flexibility matrix. The points marked by symbols show the results directly computed from the values in table 1. Also shown are continuous curves on a fine mesh of points with interpolated points. The regions are scala vestibuli (SV), scala tympani (ST), the tunnel between the arches (T), the outer hair cell region (OHC), and the layer between tectorial membrane and recticular lamina (STML). Because of the extreme flexibility of the Hensen cells, there is little difference between the flexibility of SV and OHC regions. The oscillation in the curve for the inner sulcus (IS) flexibility probably indicates that values are not interpolated adequately.

Thus the frequencies as a function of wave number can be readily determined. From these the inverse relation of wave number as a function of frequency can be determined numerically. Finally, the viscosity of the fluid is included in H and the solution of the complete system (eq. 9) determined by iteration. Generally the convergence to the complex wave number is rapid when beginning with the undamped value. Equation 9 also provides the vectors of pressure and area displacement of the fluid regions. The condition on the amplitudes of each vectors as a function of the distance x is obtained from the condition of reciprocity:

$$P_R^T \cdot V_R/n = \text{constant} \qquad (11)$$

For inviscid fluid and for traveling waves, this condition assures no loss in energy.

With this approach, the full details of the organ of Corti can be included. Subsequently, the problem can be reduced with the consideration of a few of the fluid regions, or for a full treatment, the full matrix (eq. 1) and full version of the fluid matrix (eq. 7) may be used directly. So with the same basic formulation, solutions with different degrees of complexity may be obtained.

Results

The direct calculation of the flexibility matrix (eq. 1) from the values in table 1 is carried out by Fast4. To give an indication of the results, each of the 22 diagonal coefficients of F is shown in figure 10 as a function of the distance from the stapes. An interpolation is then done on the flexibility coefficients to obtain the flexibility values on a fine mesh of points. The coefficients of the reduced flexibility matrix (eq. 4) are shown in figure 11. The values from the interpolation are shown by the continuous curves, while the values directly from table 1 are indicated by the point symbols and connected by straight lines. For the inner sulcus region (IS), a spurious oscillation occurs. So improved interpolation is needed, or more points in table 1.

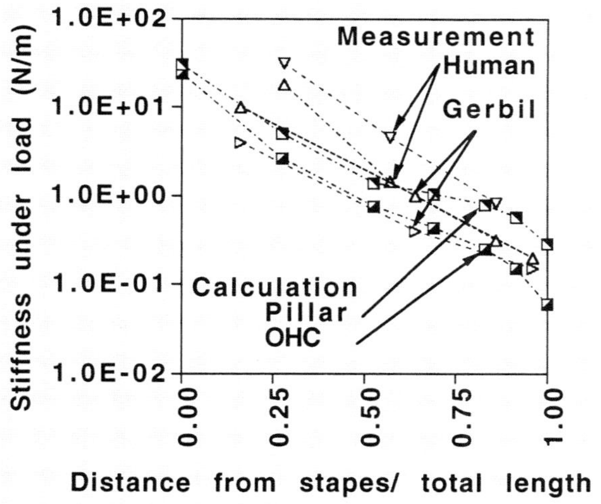

Fig. 12. Stiffness under probe of diameter 10 μm on the basilar membrane. Calculations are for buffalo cochlea, with dimensions from Tiedeman [35]. The two curves are for the stiffness for the probe located at the outer pillar, while the lower curve is for the probe at abut the third outer hair cell. Measurements are from Naidu and Mountain [17] for gerbil and from Békésy [1] for human, also showing the values at the pillars and at the outer hair cells.

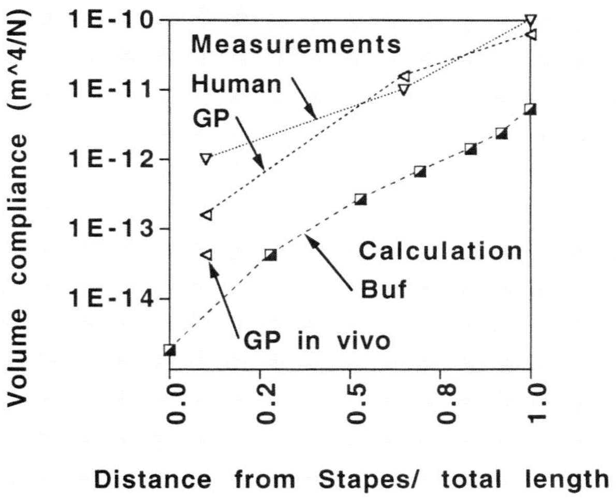

Fig. 13. Volume compliance of basilar membrane (area displacement per unit pressure). Calculations are for the buffalo cochlea, with dimensions from Tiedeman [35]. Measurements are from Békésy [1] for guinea pig and human. The in vivo measurement of the guinea pig by Dancer and Franke [7] is also shown. Flexibility of the primary sprial osseous lamina is not included in calculations, which will increase the compliance.

The total flexibility matrix (eq. 1) also yields the static stiffness of the partition under a probe 10 μm in diameter. The results of loading of the basilar membrane, from the ST side, at the outer pillar and at the third outer hair cell are shown in figure 12. The comparison with the recent mesurements by Naidu and Mountain [17] for the gerbil are amazing. Their results are normalized for a 12.5-mm length of the gerbil cochlea. Absolutely no adjustment to the values in table 1 has been made to improve this correlation. Why the 36-mm buffalo cochlea and the 12.5 mm gerbil cochlea would have such similar stiffness is open to discussion, although the frequency ranges of these two cochleas are probably about the same, and the dimensions of the basilar membrane seem to be similar. For interest, the point load values from Békésy [1] (replotted) for human are added to figure 12. Since his specimen was not fresh, his quantitative values are not to be taken as definitive. It is interesting, however, that roughly the same trend is found. Furthermore, the higher stiffness, by roughly a factor of 2, at the outer pillar than in the center of the pectinate zone is found. Also Rossi [24] and Miller [16] find this in the basal region of a fresh guinea pig cochlea. The point load values for the guinea pig are lower than for the gerbil, which can be attributed to the thinner basilar membrane in the guinea pig.

The correlation between the calculated volume compliance of the partition and Békésy's measurements shown in figure 13 is not as good. The trend is the same but the calculated values are an order of magnitude stiffer. The in vivo measurements of Dancer and Franke [7] are lower than Békésy's postmortem measurements. This seems to be consistent with the difference in the basilar membrane dimensions. The difference is also due to the fact that the flexibility of the primary spiral osseous lamina is not taken into consideration in the present calculation. Békésy mentions that the deformation of the primary is noticeable. For the buffalo the end of the bone is a substantial distance from the inner pillar, so the flexibility of the bone and the soft tissue extension will be substantial. As discussed in Taber and Steele [34], the flexibility

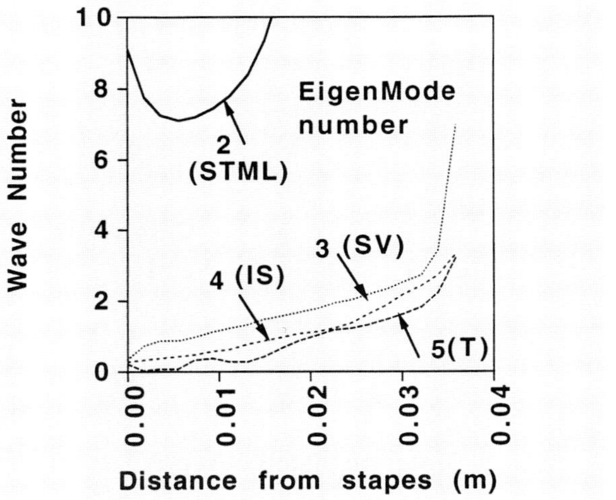

Fig. 14. Wave numbers of eigenmodes of wave propagation as a function of distance along the cochlea for the frequency 1 kHz. Eigenmode 2 is primarly a wave with significant pressure and fluid displacement in the subtectorial membrane-recticular lamina region (STML). Toward the apex, eigenmode 3 as significant and out-of-phase pressure and fluid displacement in scala vestibuli and scala tympani, corresponding to the 'normal' wave in cochlear models. Toward the apex, eigenmodes 4 and 5 correspond to significant pressure and fluid displacement in the inner sulcus (IS) and the tunnel (T) regions. Through most of the length, however, the behavior of modes 3, 4, and 5 switch several times. The wave number shown is dimensionless; however, the value of 10 gives a wavelength of about 1 mm, which normally is around the maximum amplitude in a passive model.

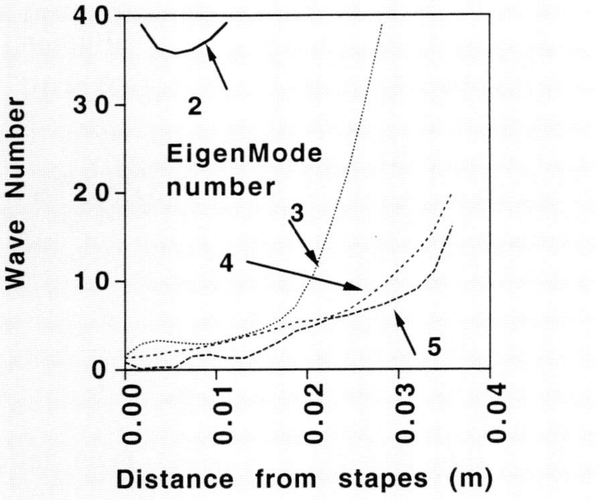

Fig. 15. Wave numbers for eigenmodes of wave propagation as a function of distance along the cochlea for the frequency 5 kHz.

of the primary has a significant effect on the long wavelength portion of the response, but little effect on the short wavelengths near CF.

At each distance, equation 10 yields eigenfrequencies for each wave number. Since a pressure vector in equation 3 with each element equal produces zero displacement of the regions, the matrix F_R has a zero eigenvalue. Thus equation 10 has one infinite eigenfrequency, which corresponds to the compression wave in the cochlea without displacement of the organ of Corti. Remaining are five eigenfrequencies that yield traveling wave modes. These are classified by eigenmode numbers 1–5 in order of the magnitude of the frequency, with the value 1 for the highest frequency. The highest seems to correspond to a very long wavelength mode associated with the motion of the cells of Hensen. The next step is to obtain numerically the inverse relation for the wave number as a function of the frequency. The results are shown in figures 14–18. For each frequency, the modes 3–5 are rather close in the basal region, then split apart as the wavelength becomes short. In the latter region, the interpretation of the modes is clear. Mode 3 corresponds to the normal mode in cochlear models, with about equal pressure and fluid displacement in scala vestibuli and scala tympani. Mode 4 corresponds to a significant activity in the inner sulcus, such as included in Steele and Lim [32]. Mode 5 corresponds to significant activity in the tunnel between the pillars. An interesting is that the interpretation of the modes associated with the eigenmode numbers switch in the basal region, particularly at the regions where the curves come close together. Part of the switching may be due to the spurious oscillation in the compliance (fig. 11). Also the strength of mode 5 is exaggerated by the condition of no leaking of fluid through the outer pillars. Nevertheless, some of switching is expected to remain with improved calculations. The points of such switching are generally referred to as transition points. So for the complete analysis taking into account the end conditions on the cochlea

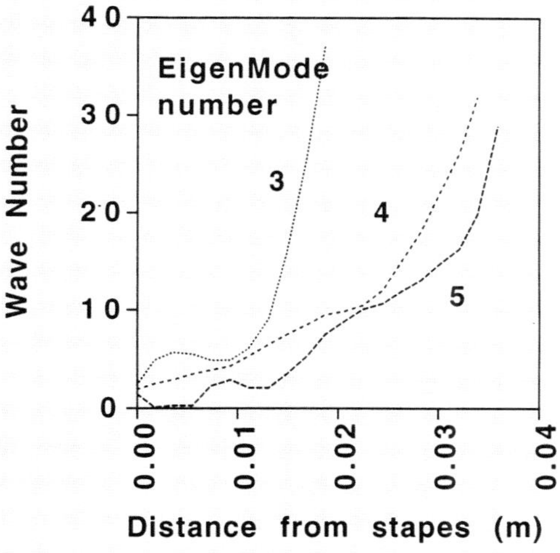

Fig. 16. Wave numbers for eigenmodes of wave propagation as a function of distance along the cochlea for the frequency 9 kHz.

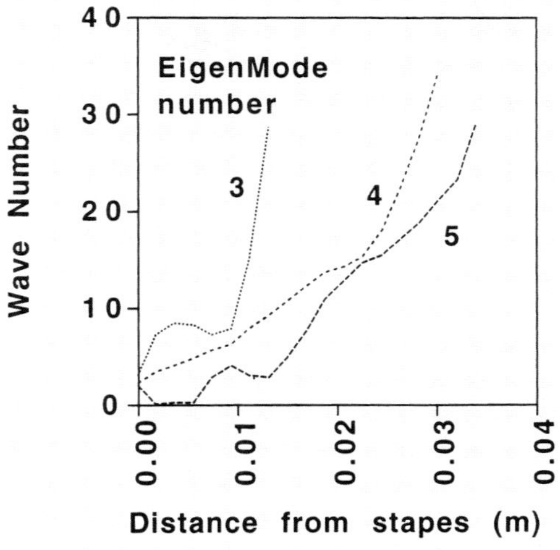

Fig. 17. Wave numbers for eigenmodes of wave propagation as a function of distance along the cochlea for the frequency 13 kHz.

and obtaining the relative size of the different modes, the procedure in Steele and Shad [29] is required.

When the fluid viscosity is included, it is expected that the maximum amplitude for a given mode will occur when the wavelength is roughly 1 mm, corresponding to a value of dimensionless wave number of 10. For example in figure 15 for 5 kHz, the eigenmode 2 will disappear and mode 3 will have a maximum at about 20 mm, the normal CF. However, modes 4 and 5 will continue apically to about 30 mm. Thus it appears that a usual cochlear map will be obtained, except that the 1-kHz results in figure 14 extend too far apically. From figure 12, it appears that the computed stiffness in the apical region may be too high.

The deformation of the cross section at the different distances from the stapes is shown in figures 19–23. The buffalo organ of Corti is remarkable for the size of the inner sulcus covered by a long tectorial membrane.

Conclusion

Considerable progress has been made and much information gained on models of the cochlea with substantial simplification of the actual details. We have outlined an

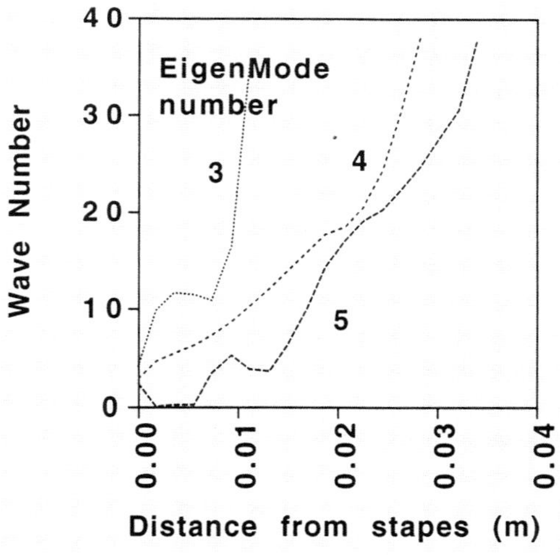

Fig. 18. Wave numbers for eigenmodes of wave propagation as a function of distance along the cochlea for the frequency 17 kHz.

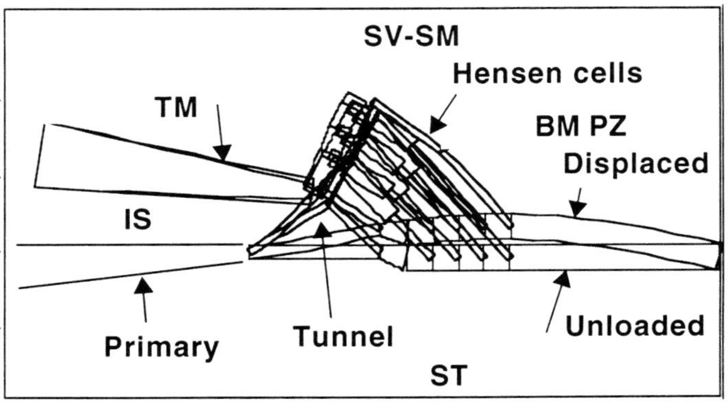

Fig. 19. Buffalo cochlea at 10 mm, with main propagating, 10 kHz, with pressures in SV and ST almost equal in magnitude and opposite in sign. The double lines show the organ in the initial unloaded and in the displaced states. For this mode, the pressure in the tunnel region is 2 times larger than that in SV. For the present calculations the primary spiral osseus lamina is rigid, with the basilar membrane clamped to the edge. The right edge of the basilar membrane is hinged. The left edge of the tectorial membrane is clamped to the limbus. The Hensen cells are only roughly approximated.

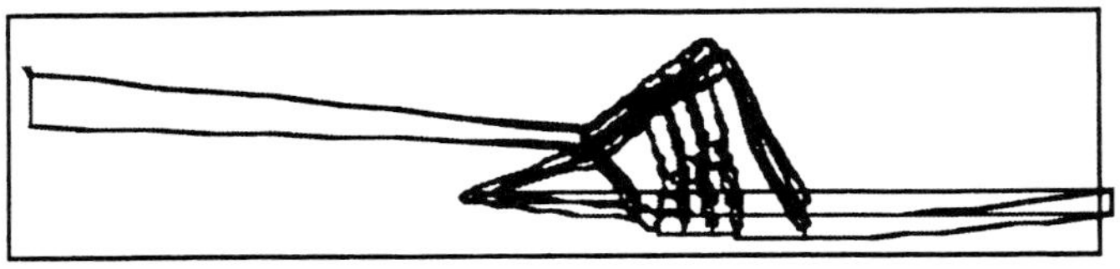

Fig. 20. Buffalo cochlea at 19 mm, with main propagating wave, 3.7 kHz, with pressures in SV and ST almost equal in magnitude and opposite in sign.

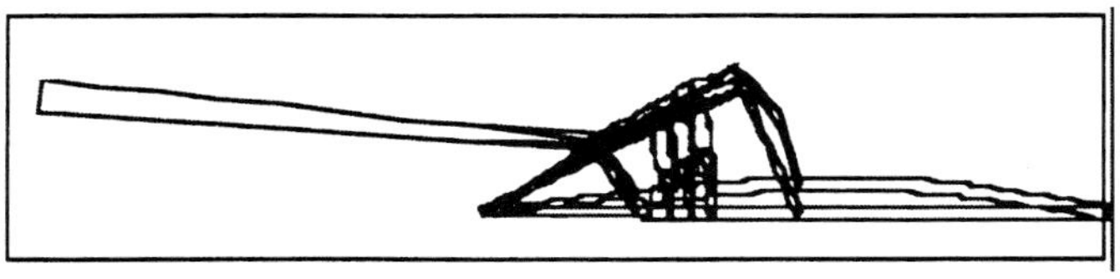

Fig. 21. Buffalo cochlea at 25 mm, with main propagating wave, 2.06 kHz, with pressures in SV and ST almost equal in magnitude and opposite in sign. For this mode, the pressure in the tunnel region is 10 times larger than that in SV.

approach with which the full three-dimensional details for the elastic structure and the three-dimensional viscous fluid can be included. The two important features are that the input required for such calculations requires only a table of the geometric and material parameters (table 1) and that the computation can be carried out in a reasonable amount of time, minutes on a laptop computer for the linear response to a single frequency. To accomplish this, reductions are made to reduce the continuum to a small arrays of the significant pressure and displacement parameters. The preliminary results indicate that several traveling waves are present and that the pressures in the inner fluid regions of the organ of Corti can be large. We expect that new features will be in store with the complete solution that do not appear in the simple models. The seemingly good values of the calculated stiffness of the basilar membrane show that it is possible to compute stiffness when the anatomy is known, including the geometry and the protein fiber type and content. We conclude that such details as in table 1 for the cochleas of greater interest will make it possible to go forward.

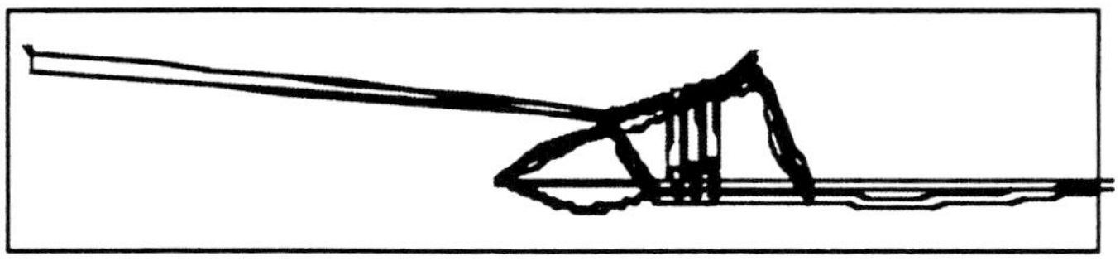

Fig. 22. Buffalo cochlea at 30 mm, with main propagating wave, 1.6 kHz, with pressures in SV and ST almost equal in magnitude and opposite in sign. For this mode, the pressure in the tunnel region is 100 times larger than that in SV.

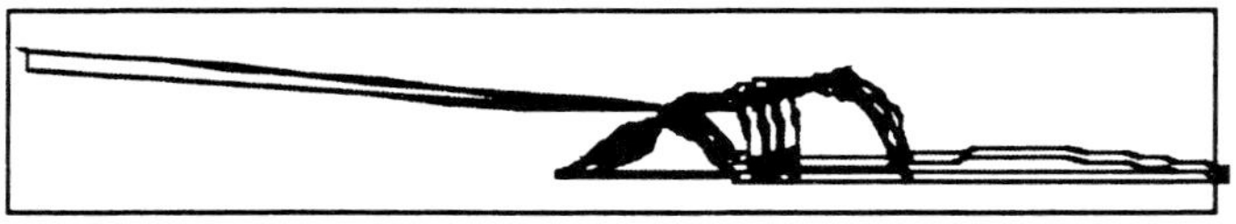

Fig. 23. Buffalo cochlea at 33 mm, with main propagating wave, 1.5 kHz, with pressures in SV and ST almost equal in magnitude and opposite in sign. For this mode, the pressure in the tunnel region is 100 times larger than that in SV. From the dimensions given by Tiedemann, the tectorial membrane is unusually long in the apical region.

References

1 von Békésy G: Experiments in Hearing. New York, McGraw-Hill, 1960.
2 de Boer E: The sulcus connection. On a mode of participation of outer hair cells in cochlear mechanics. J Acoust Soc Am 1993;93:2845–2859.
3 Böhnke F, von Mikusch-Buchberg J, Arnold W: 3D Finite Elemente Modell des cochleären Verstärkers. Biomed Tech 1996;42:311–312.
4 Boulet JAM: The role of the inner sulcus in cochlear mechanics; thesis, Stanford 1983.
5 Cabezudo LM: The ultrastructure of the basilar membrane in the cat. Acta Otolaryngol 1978; 86:160–175.
6 Chadwick RS, Dimitriades EK: The inverse problem for waves in a two sub-partition cochlear model suggests axial electromechanical coupling of outer hair cells, in Lewis ER, Long GR, Lyon RF, Narins PM, Steele CR, Hect-Poiner E (eds): Diversity in Auditory Mechanics. River Edge/NJ, World Scientific, 1996, pp 49–56.
7 Dancer A, Franke R: Intracochlear sound pressure measurements in guinea pigs. Hear Res 1980;2:191–205.
8 Fuhrmann E, Schneider W, Schultz M: Wave propagation in the cochlea (inner ear): Effects of Reissner's membrane and non-rectangular cross section. Acta Mech 1987;70:15–30.
9 Geisler CD, Sang C: A cochlear model using feed-forward outer-hair-cell forces. Hear Res 1995;85:132–146.
10 Gummer AW, Hemmert W, Zenner HP: Resonant tectorial membrane motion in the inner ear: Its crucial role in frequency tuning. Proc Natl Acad Sci USA 1996;93:8727–8732.
11 Helle R: Beobachtungen an Hydromechanischen Modellen des Innenohres mit Nachbildung von Basilarmembran, Corti-Organ, and Deckmembran; Diss, München 1974.
12 van Hengel PWJ: Emissions from cochlear modelling; thesis, Groningen, 1996.
13 Khanana SM, Flock Å, Ulfendahl M: Comparison of the tuning of outer hair cells and the basilar membrane in the isolated cochlea. Acta Otolaryngol Suppl (Stockh) 1989;467:141–156.
14 Kolston PJ, Ashmore JF: Finite element micromechanical modeling of the cochlea in three dimensions. J Acoust Soc Am 1996;99:455–467.
15 Lim KM, Steele CR: Transient response for cochlear model with 3-D fluid and feed-forward. Pan American Congress on Applied Mechanics VI, Rio de Janeiro, Jan 4–8, 1999.
16 Miller CE: Structural implications of basilar membrane compliance measurements. J Acoust Soc Am 1985;77:1765–1474.
17 Naidu RC, Mountain DC: Measurements of the stiffness map challenge a basic tenet of cochlear theories. Hear Res 1998;124:124–131.
18 Olson ES: Observing middle and inner ear mechanics with novel intracochlear pressure sensors. J Acoust Soc Am 1998;103:3445–3463.
19 Preyer S, Renz S, Hemmert W, Zenner H, Gummer A: Receptor potential of outer hair cells isolated from base to apex of adult guinea-pig cochlea: Implications for cochlear tuning mechanisms. Audit Neurosci 1996;2:145–157.
20 Raftenberg MN: Flow of endolymph in the inner spiral sulcus and the subtectorial space. J Acoust Soc Am 1990;87:2606–2620.
21 Ranke OF: Theory of operation of the cochlea: A contribution to the hydrodynamics of the cochlea. J Acoust Soc Am 1950;22:772–777.
22 Recio A, Rich NC, Narayan SS, Ruggero MA: Basilar-membrane responses to clicks at the base of the chinchilla cochlea. J Acoust Soc Am 1998;103:1972–1989.
23 Ruggero MA, Rich NC, Recio A, Narayan SS, Robles L: Basilar-membrane responses to tones at the base of the chinchilla cochlea. J Acoust Soc Am 1997;101:2151–2163.
24 Rossi GT: Basilar membrane compliance variations in the arcuate and pectinate zones. Eng. thesis, Stanford University, Stanford CA, 1983.
25 Siebert WM: Ranke revisited – A simple short-wave cochlear model. J Acoust Soc Am 1974; 56:594–600.
26 Steele CR: Behavior of the basilar membrane with pure tone excitation. J Acoust Soc Am 1974;55:148–162.
27 Steele CR: Cochlear mechanics; in Skalak R, Chien S (eds): Handbook of Bioengineering. New York, McGraw-Hill, 1987, pp 30.11–30.22
28 Steele CR, Baker G, Tolomeo JA, Zetes DE: Electro-mechanical models of the outer hair cell; in Duifhuis H, Horst JW, van Dijk P, van Netten SM (eds): Biophysics of Hair Cell Sensory Systems. River Edge/NJ, World Scientific, 1993.
29 Steele CR, Shad KR: Asymptotic-numeric solution for shells of revolution. Appl Mech Rev 1995;48:part 2.
30 Steele CR, Baker GA, Tolomeo JA, Zetes DE: Cochlear mechanics; in Schneck DJ (ed): Biomechanics Section. CRC Biomedical Engineering Handbook, ed 2. Boca Raton, CRC Press, 1999.
31 Steele CR: Three-dimensional computation of the cochlea; in Lewis ER, Long GR, Lyon RF, Narins PM, Steele CR, Hect-Poiner E (eds): Diversity in Auditory Mechanics. River Edge/NJ, World Scientific, 1997, pp 455–461.
32 Steele CR, Lim KM: Cochlear model with 3-D fluid, inner sulcus, and feed-forward mechanism. Audiol Neurootol 1999;4:197–203.
33 Taber LA, Steele CR: Comparison of 'WKB' and experimental results for three-dimensional cochlear models: J Acoust Soc Am 1979;65:1007–1018.
34 Taber LA, Steele CR: A cochlear model including three-dimensional fluid and four modes of partition flexibility. J Acoust Soc Am 1981;70:426–436.
35 Tiedemann H: A new approach to theory of hearing. Acta Otolaryngol Suppl 1970;277:1–50.
36 Zhang L, Mountain DC, Hubbard AE: Shape changes from base to apex cannot predict characteristics frequency changes. Diversity in Auditory Mechanics. Berkeley, University of California, 1996, pp 611–618.
37 Zhou G, Bintz L, Anderson DZ, Bright KE: A life-sized physical model of the human cochlea with optical holographic readout. J Acoust Soc Am 1994;93:1516–1523.

ORL

ORL 1999;61:252–258

Effect of Irregularities in Basilar Membrane Impedance on TEOAEs: Theoretical Considerations

Hiroshi Wada[a] Takaya Nakajima[a] Kenji Ohyama[b]

[a]Department of Mechanical Engineering, Tohoku University and [b]Tohoku Ro-sai Hospital, Sendai, Japan

Key Words
Transiently evoked otoacoustic emissions · Irregularities · Basilar membrane · Outer hair cell motility · One-dimensional model of a cochlea · Theoretical consideration

Abstract
Transiently evoked otoacoustic emissions (TEOAEs) are believed to be attributed to the presence of impedance discontinuities on the basilar membrane in the cochlea. However, the generation mechanism of TEOAEs has not been clarified. In this study, using the mathematical model of a cochlea, which has the impedance discontinuities on the basilar membrane, TEOAEs were simulated. The results reveal that the TEOAEs are produced by not only the active process associated with the outer hair cell motility, but also the presence of impedance discontinuities at a site of the basilar membrane whose characteristic frequency is close to the stimulus frequency. Therefore, it may be said that the TEOAEs in response to a tone burst stimulus reflect the condition at the specific point of the cochlea.

Introduction

Otoacoustic emissions (OAEs) evoked by a transient acoustic stimulus such as a click or a tone burst are called transiently evoked OAEs (TEOAEs). A typical measurement result of TEOAEs waveforms is shown in figure 1. Two wave trains are clearly seen at about 11 and 16 ms after the onset of the stimulus, and these are termed as the fast and slow components of TEOAEs [1].

In recent papers, several authors mention that TEOAEs would be attributed to the presence of impedance discontinuities on the basilar membrane (BM) in the cochlea [2–4]. The longitudinal stiffness of the BM has been observed to be much smaller than its transverse stiffness, because the fibrils in the BM are arranged in radial and spiral directions [5]. As a result, the BM impedance is thought to be structural irregularities in a longitudinal direction by the discontinuities arrangement of the fibrils in transverse direction. The discontinuities of outer hair cell (OHC) rows are thought to be another factor of the BM impedance discontinuities [6–8]. However, it has not been clear whether the TEOAEs are generated by the BM impedance discontinuities. Therefore, in this study, using the one-dimensional mathematical model of the cochlea [9], an attempt is made to clarify the generation mechanism of the TEOAEs.

KARGER

Fax + 41 61 306 12 34
E-Mail karger@karger.ch
www.karger.com

© 1999 S. Karger AG, Basel
0301–1569/99/0615–0252$17.50/0

Accessible online at:
http://BioMedNet.com/karger

Hiroshi Wada
Department of Mechanical Engineering, Tohoku University
Aoba-yama 01, Sendai 980-8579 (Japan)
Tel. +81 22 217 6938, Fax +81 22 217 6939
E-Mail wada@cc.mech.tohoku.ac.jp

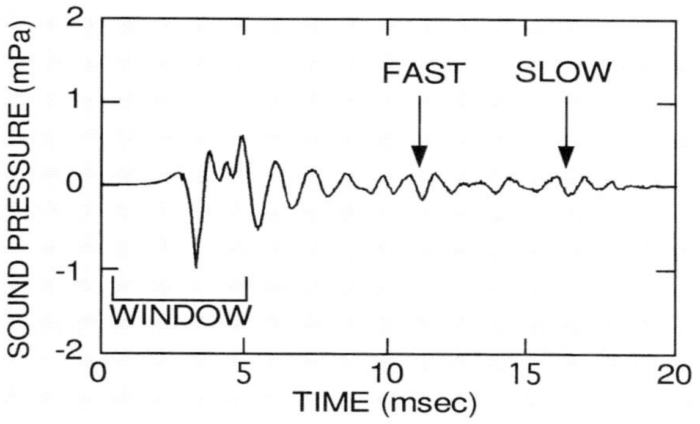

Fig. 1. A typical measurement result of TEOAEs waveforms. Tone burst signals of 3 ms in duration with 1 ms rise and fall time, 1.0 kHz in frequency and 60 dBpeSPL in level are applied. The response window is set at 0–10 ms. The fast and slow components are clearly seen at the latency of 11 and 16 ms.

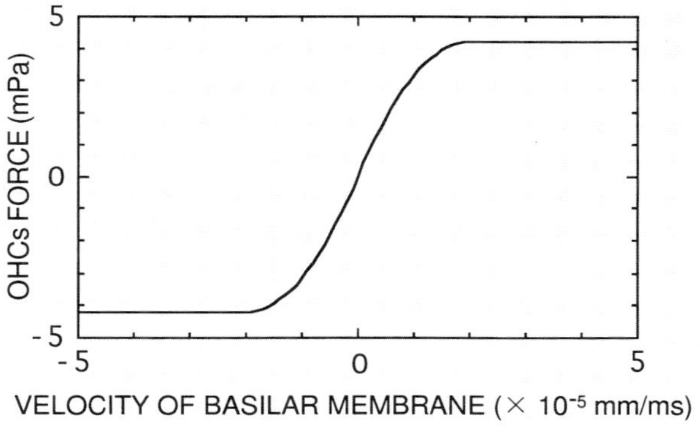

Fig. 2. Relationship between the force of the OHCs and the velocity of the BM at the position corresponding to the CF of 1.0 kHz. The OHCs force is saturated when the BM velocity is large.

Theoretical Analysis

If a partition of the BM is assumed to be a vibration system with one degree of freedom, the equation of the BM motion is given by

$$M(x)\frac{\partial^2 u(x,t)}{\partial t^2} + R(x)\frac{\partial u(x,t)}{\partial t} + K(x)u(x,t) = p(x,t) + P_{OHC}(x,t) \quad (1)$$

where x is the distance from the stapes, t is the time, $M(x)$, $R(x)$ and $K(x)$ are the mass, damping and stiffness of the BM per unit area, respectively, $u(x,t)$ is the displacement of the BM in a vertical direction to the x axis, $p(x,t)$ is the difference in pressure between the scala vestibuli and scala tympani, and $P_{OHC}(x,t)$ is the force per unit area generated by the active behavior of the OHCs. Based on the report that input-output function for an OHC shows a compressive nonlinearity [10], as shown in figure 2, the force of the OHCs is assumed to vary in conjunction with the velocity of the BM and the distance from the basal end.

In this model, in order to express irregularities in the BM impedance, an irregular function is introduced in the form

$$\delta(x) = \{1 + \delta'(x)\} \times 100, \quad (2)$$

$$\delta'(x) = \begin{cases} a_i \ (x = x_i,\ i = 1,2,3,...,n) \\ 0 \ (x \neq x_i,\ i = 1,2,3,...,n), \end{cases} \quad (3)$$

where a is the magnitude of the irregularity and x_i is the position of the irregularity [11–13]. If M_0, K_0 and R_0 represent the mass, stiffness and damping coefficient of the BM before introducing the irregularities, these after introducing the irregularities are given by

$$M(x) = M_0(x) \times \frac{\delta_M(x)}{100},$$

$$K(x) = K_0(x) \times \frac{\delta_K(x)}{100}, \quad (4)$$

$$R(x) = R_0(x) \times \frac{\delta_R(x)}{100}$$

where the subscripts M, K and R indicate the mass, stiffness and damping coefficient of the BM, respectively. If the irregular function $\delta_M(x)$ related to the BM mass is introduced such as shown in figure 3a, the BM mass distribution along the characteristic frequency (CF) axis is given as depicted in figure 3b.

TEOAEs are transmitted to the external auditory meatus through the middle ear and detected most distinctly at the middle ear resonance frequency at around 1.0 kHz. Therefore, the effect of the middle ear transmission on OAEs seems not to be negligible [14], and this effect is taken into consideration in this study. If the forward and reverse middle ear transmission factors are given by T_f and T_r, respectively, the relationship between the input pressure p_{ti} in front of the tympanic membrane and the intracochlear pressure p_{ci} in the scala vestibuli is expressed by

$$p_{ci}(t) = T_f p_{ti}(t) \quad (5)$$

and the relationship between the intracochlear pressure p_{co} generated by the cochlear amplification and the output pressure p_{to} detected as OAEs in front of the tympanic membrane is given by

$$p_{to}(t) = T_r p_{co}(t). \quad (6)$$

For the numerical calculations, the values of T_f and T_r measured by Puria and Rosowski [15] are applied.

The finite-difference method and the fourth-order Runge-Kutta method are put to use to discretize these equations in space and time. In this analysis, the cochlea is divided into 512 sections and the time step is taken to be 1/128 ms. The numerical calculations are carried out using the work station (SUN, SPARCstation20).

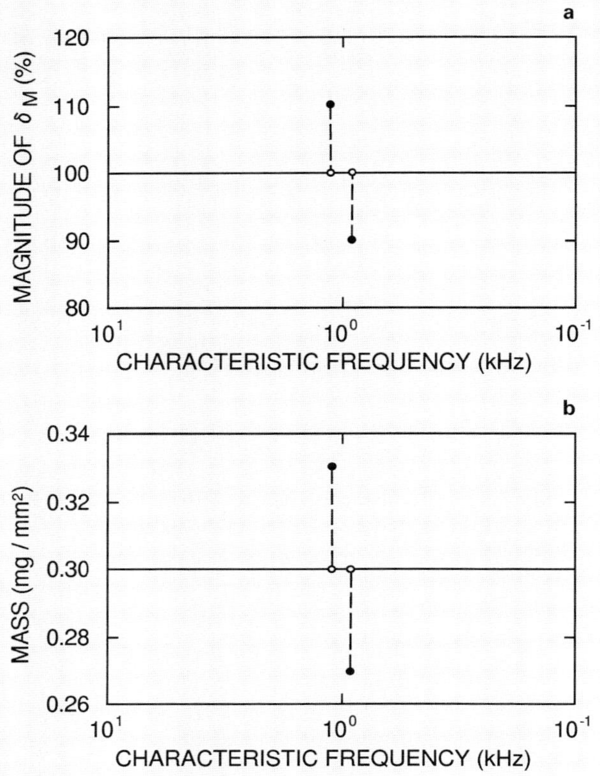

Fig. 3. Expression of the BM irregularities. **a** Irregular function $\delta_M(x)$ introduced to the BM mass versus the CF axis. At the positions corresponding to the CFs of 1.1 and 0.9 kHz, the values of $\delta_M(x)$ are 10% larger and smaller than those of other positions, respectively. **b** BM mass versus the CF axis. The BM mass corresponding to the CF of 1.1 kHz is 0.33 mg/mm^2, that to the CF of 0.9 kHz is 0.27 mg/mm^2 and that of other positions is 0.30 mg/mm^2.

Results

Figure 4 shows a numerical result of the waveforms when the motility function of the OHCs is considered to be normal along the CF axis, but the irregularities in the BM impedance are not taken into account. In this case, although the waveforms caused by the tone burst stimuli are seen until 10 ms, such TEOAEs waveforms as those displayed in figure 1 are not obtainable.

In order to understand the effect of the irregularities in the BM impedance, firstly, the irregular function $\delta_M(x)$ shown in figure 5a is introduced to the mass of the BM impedance. The magnitude of the irregularity at the single position, corresponding to the CF of 1.2 kHz, is 10% larger than that of other positions. The numerically obtained waveforms depicted in figure 5b are similar to those shown in figure 4 until 10 ms after the onset of the stimulus. However, beyond 10 ms, sinusoidal waveforms are observed. These waveforms beyond 10 ms are Fourier-transformed to the frequency domain, and the result is shown in figure 5c. The spectrum has a prominent peak at the frequency of 1.2 kHz, and this frequency is coincident with the CF corresponding to the BM position where the irregularity is introduced. This agreement is also obtained when the irregularities are introduced to the stiffness and damping of the BM impedance.

Figure 6 shows the relationship between the peak-to-peak amplitude of the waveforms beyond 10 ms and the CF corresponding to the BM position when the stimulus is the same as those in figures 1, 4, and 5. The magnitude of the irregularity at the corresponding position is 10% larger than those of other positions in figure 6a, and 10% smaller in figure 6b. The results reveal that the peak-to-peak amplitude of the waveforms is largest when the irregularity is introduced at the position where the corresponding CF is 1.0 kHz, and that the effect of the damping on the amplitude is smaller than those of the mass and stiffness.

Figure 7 shows the waveforms when the irregularities are introduced at the two positions. The dashed line is obtained by combining linearly the waveforms depicted by the fine solid line when the mass of the BM impedance at the single position, corresponding to the CF of 0.9 kHz, is 10% larger than those of other positions, with the waveforms given by the fine dashed line when its stiffness at the single position, corresponding to the CF of 1.2 kHz, is 10% smaller than those of other positions. The solid line is obtained when the irregularities are introduced simultaneously at the same two positions and with the same amplitude as the cases shown by the fine solid and dashed lines. The solid line coincides with the dashed line. Coincidence is also obtainable even when a combination of the other different irregularities, e.g. the stiffness and damping irregularities, is introduced. This result implies that the waveforms induced by introducing the irregularities of the BM impedance at more than two positions, are obtainable by combining linearly the waveforms induced by introducing the irregularity at one position with each other.

The relationship between the waveforms and irregularities shown in figures 5–7 leads to a possibility of producing TEOAEs waveforms by introducing appropriate irregularities. Although there are a lot of combinations of the mass, stiffness and damping of the BM impedance, as an example, the irregularity functions $\delta_M(x)$ and $\delta_K(x)$ shown in fig-

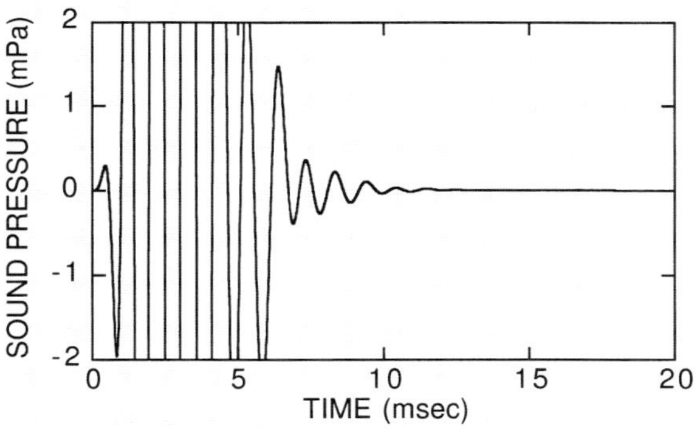

4

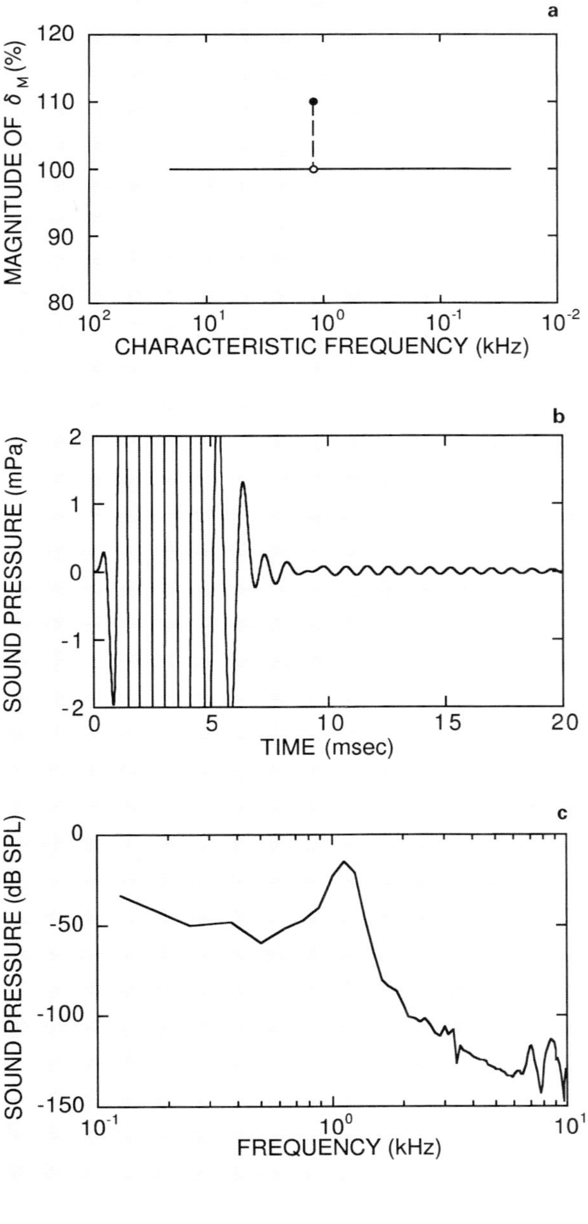

5

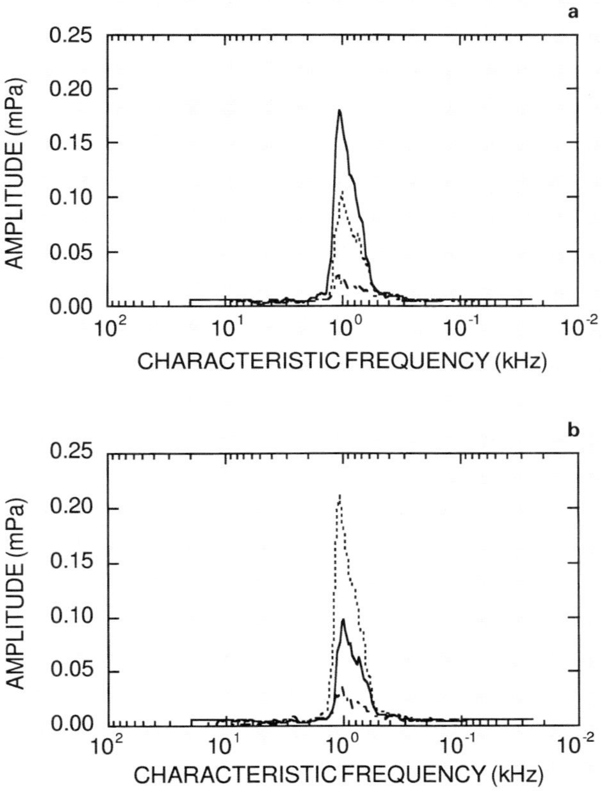

6

Fig. 4. Numerically obtained waveforms when the OHCs active behavior is considered to be normal, but the irregularities of the BM impedance are not taken into account. The stimulus is the same as that in figure 1. Such TEOAEs waveforms as those shown in figure 1 are not obtainable.

Fig. 5. Numerical result when the irregularity in the BM impedance is introduced at the single position. **a** The irregular function $\delta_M(x)$ introduced to the BM mass versus the CF axis. The magnitude of the irregularity at the single position, corresponding to the CF of 1.2 kHz, is 10% larger than that of other positions. **b** Numerically obtained waveforms. The stimulus is the same as those in figures 1 and 4. Beyond 10 ms, sinusoidal waveforms are observed. **c** Fourier-transformed spectrum of the waveforms shown in **b** beyond 10 ms. The spectrum has a prominent peak at the frequency of 1.2 kHz, and this frequency is coincident with the CF corresponding to the BM position where the irregularity is introduced.

Fig. 6. Relationship between the peak-to-peak amplitude of the waveforms beyond 10 ms and the CF corresponding to the BM position where the irregularity is introduced. The stimulus is the same as those in the previous figures. **a** Introduction of the 10% larger BM irregularity. **b** Introduction of the 10% smaller BM irregularity. **a**, **b** —— = mass; – – – = stiffness; –·–·– = damping. The amplitude is largest when the irregularity is introduced at the position where the corresponding CF coincides with the stimulus frequency. The effect of the damping on the amplitude is smaller than those of the mass and stiffness.

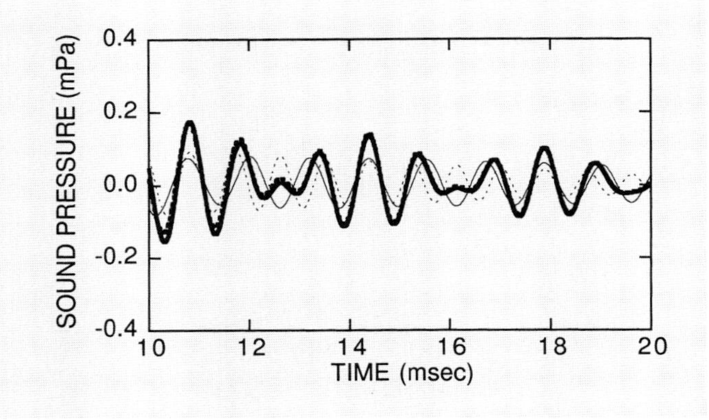

7

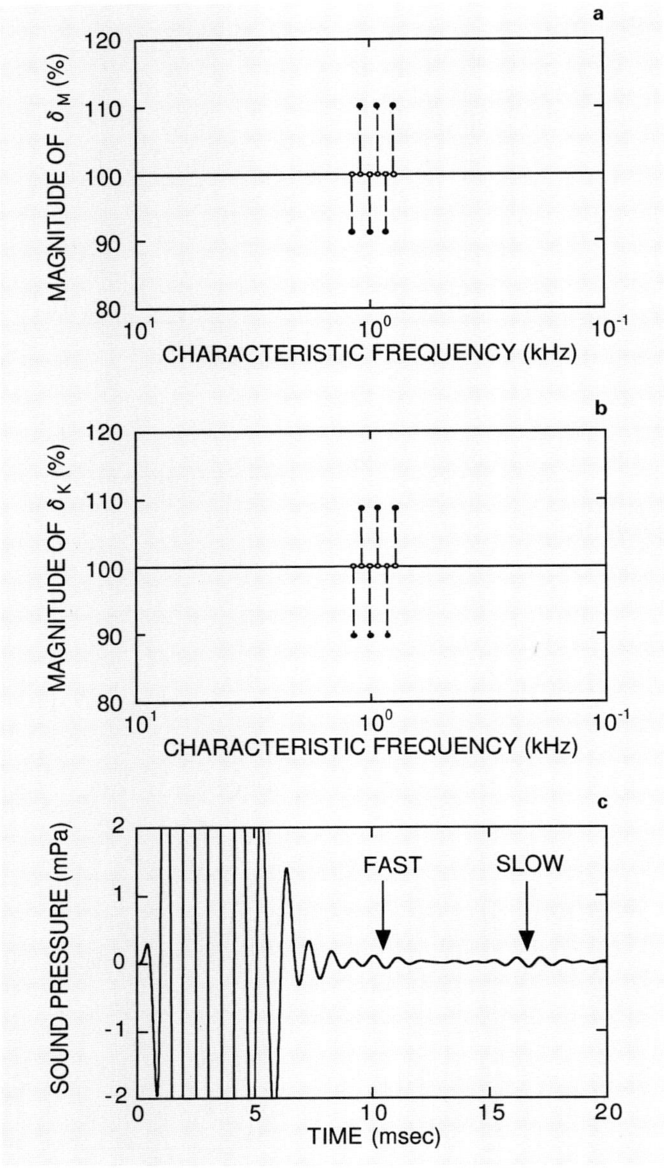

8

Fig. 7. Numerically obtained waveforms. The stimulus is the same as those in the previous figures. —— = The BM mass at the single position, corresponding to the CF of 0.9 kHz, is 10% larger than those of other positions; – – – = the BM stiffness at the single position, corresponding to the CF of 1.2 kHz, is 10% smaller than those of other positions; ▪▪▪▪▪ = the waveforms obtained by combining linearly the waveforms depicted by the fine solid line with those by the fine dashed line; ▬ = the waveforms obtained by introducing the BM irregularities simultaneously at the same two positions and with the same amplitude as the cases shown by the fine solid and dashed lines. The solid line coincides with the dashed line.

Fig. 8. Numerical result when the irregularities in the BM impedance are introduced. **a** The irregular function $\delta_M(x)$ introduced to the BM mass versus the CF axis. The irregularities are given at the interval of 80 Hz at around the CF of 1.0 kHz. The amplitude of the irregularities is 10% larger or smaller than that of other positions. **b** The irregular function $\delta_K(x)$ introduced to the BM stiffness versus the CF axis. The condition of the irregularities is the same as that given in **a**. **c** Numerically obtained waveforms. The stimulus is the same as those in the previous figures. This result resembles the measurement one shown in figure 1, and the two wave trains are noticeable at about 10 and 16 ms after the onset of the stimulus.

ures 8a and b are considered. In this case, the waveforms depicted in figure 8c are induced. These numerically obtained waveforms resemble the actual measurement result shown in figure 1, and the two wave trains are noticeable at about 10 and 16 ms after the onset of the stimulus.

Input-output curves of the fast and slow components of the measurement and numerical results are depicted in figure 9. In this case, the curve of the fast component is steeper than that of the slow component. Figure 10 shows the relationship between the amplitude of the fast and slow components and the force of the entire BM position along the x axis generated by the OHCs motility. The amplitude decreases with a decrease in the force, in other words, with a decrease in the amplitude shown in figure 2. Moreover, the decreasing ratio of the slow component is much larger than that of the fast component.

In order to investigate the effect of the OHCs force at the specific BM position on the TEOAEs, the two states of the OHCs force are considered. One state is to weaken the OHCs force at the position, corresponding to the CF of 1.0 kHz, which is depicted by the solid line in figure 11a, and the other state is to weaken the OHCs force along the

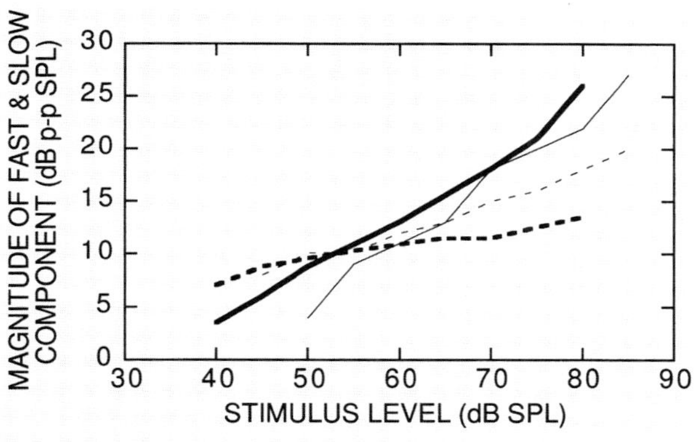

9

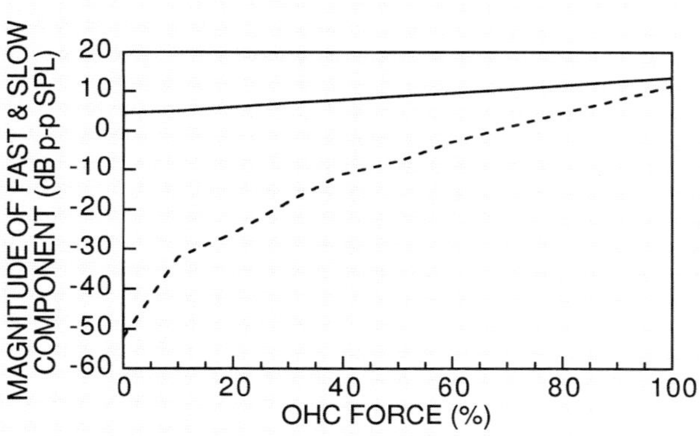

10

Fig. 9. Numerical and measurement input-output curves of the fast and slow components. ▬ = Numerically obtained fast component; ▪▪▪▪▪ = numerically obtained slow component; —— = measured fast component; – – – = measured slow component. The introduced irregular functions are the same as those shown in figure 8. The stimulus is the same as those in previous figures. The numerical results are similar to the measurement ones, and the curves of the fast components are steeper than those of the slow components.

Fig. 10. Relationship between the amplitude of the fast and slow components and the force generated by the OHCs motility. —— = Fast component; – – – = slow component. The force is assumed to be generated by the OHCs motility at the entire BM position along the x axis. The introduced irregular functions are the same as those shown in figure 8, and the stimulus is also the same as those in the previous figures. The decreasing ratio of the slow component is much larger than that of the fast component.

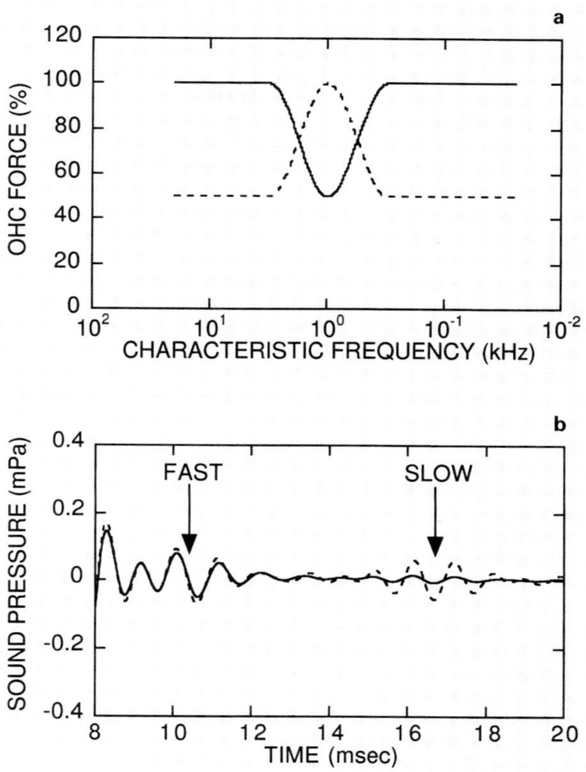

Fig. 11. Effect of the OHCs force at the specific BM position on the TEOAEs waveforms. **a** OHCs force versus the CF axis. —— = The OHCs force at the BM position, corresponding to the CF of 1.0 kHz, is weakened to 50% of the OHCs force at other positions; – – – = the OHCs force along the x axis is weakened to 50% except for the position corresponding to the CF of 1.0 kHz. **b** Numerically obtained waveforms. The introduced irregular functions are the same as those shown in figure 8, and the stimulus is also the same as those in the previous figures. —— = Obtained by the assumption of the solid line of **a**; – – – = obtained by the assumption of the dashed line of **a**. The slow component of the TEOAEs is not generated when the assumption of the solid line of **a** is applied.

x axis, except for the position, corresponding to the CF of 1.0 kHz, which is depicted by the dashed line in figure 11a. In both states, the same condition of the irregularities of the BM impedance as shown in figures 8a and b is applied. The result given in figure 11b reveals that the slow component of the TEOAEs is not generated in the former case.

Discussion

When the irregularities in the BM impedance are not introduced, even if the OHCs force acts on the BM normally, the TEOAEs waveforms are not obtainable. By contrast, when the irregularity is introduced at the single position of the BM, the sinusoidal waveforms, whose frequency is coincident with the CF corresponding to the irregularity position of the BM, are produced beyond 10 ms after the onset of the stimulus. The generation mechanism of the sinusoidal waveforms is speculated as follows: The traveling waves move forward along the BM from the basal end toward the apical end. When the traveling waves arrive at the irregular position, some of them reflect because of the discontinuity of the BM impedance. They move backward, and reflect again at the basal end. A repeat of the reflections at the irregular position of the BM and the basal end generates such sinusoidal waves as shown in figure 5b. The amplitude of the sinusoidal waveforms beyond 10 ms increases when the introduced irregular position of the BM approaches to the position, whose corresponding CF coincides with the stimulus frequency, and the amplitude is largest when the corresponding CF is coincident with the stimulus frequency.

When the irregularities of the BM impedance are introduced at more than two points, a combination of the respective reflected waves may produce the waveforms beyond 10 ms. Even if other combinations of the irregularities in the BM impedance other than those shown in figure 8a and b are applied, TEOAEs will be generated. However, as shown in figure 11, in spite of taking account of the irregularities of the BM impedance, if the OHCs activity is weak at around the position, whose corresponding CF is close to the stimulus frequency, the slow component of the TEOAEs is not generated.

As shown in references 1 and 9, the slow component has a lower threshold than the fast component, and the input-output curve of the former is slower in gradient than that of the latter. The numerical results shown in figure 9 have the same tendency as those reported by Tanaka et al. [1] and Wada and Noguchi [9]. They also described that the slow component might be more sensitive than the fast component to the active process of the tuning mechanism in the cochlea. If it is assumed that the hearing impairment is caused by the decline of the OHCs activity, the numberical results shown in figure 10 support his description. Because of the similarities between the numerical and measurement results mentioned above, the model used in this study may be adequate to investigate the generation mechanism of TEOAEs.

The discussions so far suggest that the TEOAEs would be produced by not only the presence of the impedance discontinuities at a site of the BM, whose CF is close to the stimulus frequency, but also the active process associated with OHCs at the same site. Therefore, it may be said that the TEOAEs in response to a tone burst stimulus reflect the condition at the specific point of the cochlea, and that the level of the TEOAEs would be small in spite of the normal OHCs activity when the irregularities in the BM impedance do not properly exist.

Conclusion

Using the one-dimensional mathematical model of the cochlea, an attempt is made to clarify the generation mechanism of the TEOAEs. The results lead to the conclusion that the TEOAEs would be produced by not only the active process associated with the OHCs, but also the presence of the impedance discontinuities at a site of the BM whose CF is close to the stimulus frequency. Therefore, it may be said that the TEOAEs in response to a tone burst stimulus reflect the condition at the specific point of the cochlea.

References

1 Tanaka Y, Suzuki M, Inoue T: Evoked otoacoustic emissions in sensorineural hearing impairment: Its clinical implications. Ear Hear 1990;11:134–143.
2 Kemp DT: Stimulated acoustic emissions from within the human auditory system. J Acoust Soc Am 1978;64:1386–1391.
3 Hilger AW, Furness DN, Wilson JP: The possible relationship between transient evoked otoacoustic emissions and organ of Corti irregularities in the guinea pig. Hear Res 1995;84:1–11.
4 Fukazawa T: Evoked otoacoustic emission in a nonlinear model of the cochlea. Hear Res 1992; 59:17–24.
5 Mikuni H, Fukuda S, Kucuk B, Inuyama Y, Ushiki T, Abe K: The three-dimensional fibrillar arrangement of the basilar membrane in the mouse cochlea. Eur Arch Otorhinolaryngol 1995;252:459–498.
6 Lonsbury-Martin BL, Martin GK, Probst R, Coats AC: Spontaneous otoacoustic emissions in a nonhuman primate. II. Cochlear anatomy. Hear Res 1988;33:69–93.
7 Kim DO: Active and nonlinear cochlear biomechanics and the role of outer-hair-cell subsystem in the mammalian auditory system. Hear Res 1986;22:105–114.
8 Clark WW, Kim DO, Aurek PM, Bohne BA: Spontaneous otoacoustic emissions in chinchilla ear canals: Correlation with histopathology and suppression by external tones. Hear Res 1984;16:299–314.
9 Wada H, Noguchi S: Theoretical analysis of otoacoustic emissions; in Hayashi K, Ishikawa H (eds): Computational Biomechanics. Tokyo, Springer, 1996, pp 233–245.
10 Cody AR, Russell IJ: The response of hair cells in the basal turn of the guinea-pig cochlea to tones. J Physiol 1987;383:551–569.
11 Sun X, He N, Lam CF: Modeling the fine structure of the $2f_1$–f_2 acoustic distortion product. I. Model development. J Acoust Soc Am 1994; 96:2166–2174.
12 Sun X, He N, Lam CF: Modeling the fine structure of the $2f_1$–f_2 acoustic distortion product. II. Model evaluation. J Acoust Soc Am 1994; 96:2175–2183.
13 Wit HP, Avan P: Wavelet analysis of real ear and synthesized click evoked otoacoustic emissions. Hear Res 1994;73:141–147.
14 Wada H, Ohyama K, Kobayashi T, Sunaga N, Koike T: Relationship between evoked otoacoustic emissions and middle-ear dynamic characteristics. Audiology 1993;32:282–292.
15 Puria S, Rosowski JJ: Measurement of reverse transmission in the human middle ear: Preliminary results; in Lewis ER, Long GR, Lyon RF, Narins PM, Steele CR, Hecht-Poinar E (eds): Diversity in Auditory Mechanics. Singapore, World Scientific, 1996, pp 151–157.

ORL

ORL 1999;61:259–267

New Approach for 3D Imaging and Geometry Modeling of the Human Inner Ear

Uwe Vogel

Fraunhofer Institute for Microelectronic Circuits and Systems (IMS2), Dresden, Germany

Key Words

3D imaging · Geometry model · Temporal bone · Microtomography

Abstract

Obtaining high-resolution three-dimensional (3D) geometry data performs a necessary assumption for modeling cochlear mechanics. Preferably this procedure has to be done noninvasively to preserve the original morphology. Depending on the actual application, various levels of spatial resolution and tissue differentiation should be reached. Here a new approach is presented which allows 3D imaging of temporal bone specimens with intact regions of interest and spatial resolution currently in the 10-μm range, but providing capabilities for future enhancements down to the submicron level. The technique is based on microtomography by X-rays or synchrotron radiation respectively. The structural data are reconstructed and converted to geometry data by 3D image processing, and eventually transferred into simulation environments, e.g., Finite Element Analysis, but may also be used for general visualization tasks in research, clinics, and education.

Introduction

The availability of high-resolution, noninvasive imaging approaches for the human inner ear would serve an entire set of requests and applications in the field of otology. From a research viewpoint the knowledge of volume geometry data is a necessary assumption for modeling of sound or electrical field propagation and irritation generation inside the inner ear [1–3]. Regarding clinics, new aspects for diagnostics and therapy may be conducted, e.g., for operation planning in cochlea implantation [4–6]. For both modeling and clinics' purposes the derivation of inter- and intraindividual data is of special interest. Considering the anatomic viewpoint the time-consuming and mostly invasive procedures for investigating internal temporal bone structures could be at least partially replaced by advanced techniques. This provides three-dimensional (3D) visualizations or solid models of those objects.

Thus the goal in evaluating techniques for inner ear imaging is directed onto providing complex 3D data noninvasively, i.e., without affecting the region of interest or even applicable under in vivo and in situ conditions, and their visualization by tissue- and function-dependent differentiation of macro- and microscopic structures.

So far there are several physical techniques for structural imaging of the temporal bone. Some of them have already been used for temporal bone imaging. But most of them incorporate considerable limitations regarding the

KARGER

Fax + 41 61 306 12 34
E-Mail karger@karger.ch
www.karger.com

© 1999 S. Karger AG, Basel
0301–1569/99/0615–0259$17.50/0

Accessible online at:
http://BioMedNet.com/karger

Dipl.-Ing. Uwe Vogel
Fraunhofer Institute for Microelectronic Circuits and Systems
Grenzstrasse 28
D–01109 Dresden (Germany)
Tel. +49 351 8823 282, Fax +49 351 8823 266, E-Mail vogel@imsdd.fhg.de

Table 1. Classification and comparison of inner ear imaging techniques by their physical information carrier

Physical carrier	Technique	3D?	Spatial resolution, mm	Structure differentiation	Volume (V)/ surface (S)?	Non-invasive?	In vivo?	Imaged structures/ reference
X-rays	Plane image	2D	>0.01	Distribution of N of chemical elements	V	Yes	Yes	Labyrinth, internal ear canal [7]
	Direct magnification	2D	>0.001	Distribution of N of chemical elements	V	Yes	No	Cochlea [6]
	Conventional CT	3D	lateral: >0.1 slice: >1	Distribution of N of chemical elements	V	Yes	Yes	Labyrinth, cochlea, internal ear canal [8–10]
	Helical CT	3D	lateral: >0.1 slice: >0.3	Distribution of N of chemical elements	V	Yes	Yes	Labyrinth, cochlea, internal ear canal [4, 11–13]
	IPOM [14]	3D	>0.1	Distribution of N of chemical elements	V	Yes	Yes	(Under investigation by the author)
Synchrotron radiation	Absorption micro-CT	3D	>0.001	Distribution of refractive indices	V	Yes	No	Labyrinth, cochlea, internal ear canal [15, this paper]
	Phase-contrast micro-CT	3D	>0.001	Distribution of N of chemical elements	V	Yes	No	(Currently under evaluation by the author)
Light	Microscopy	2D, 3D	>0.0001	Staining, fluorescence	S	Limited	Limited	Various structures (in combination with histologic sectioning)
	Tomography	3D	>0.01	Staining, fluorescence	V	Limited	No	Cochlea [16, 17]
	Projection	3D	>0.01		S	Limited	No	Labyrinth [18]
Particle waves	Electron microscopy	2D, 3D	>0.0000001	Coated structures	S	No	No	Membranes, hair cells [19]
Magnetic resonance	Clinical MRT	3D	>0.3	Proton distribution, T_1, T_2	V	Yes	Yes	Cochlea, labyrinth, nerves [20–23]
	Micro-MRT	3D	>0.01	Proton distribution, T_1, T_2	V	Yes	No	Cochlea, labyrinth [24]
Other	Histologic sectioning	2D, 3D	>0.001	Staining, fluorescence	V	No	No	Various structures [25–30]

main objectives. The following survey describes different classification criteria of possible approaches for 3D imaging of internal temporal bone structures including the inner ear:

(1) *Physical imaging technique:* This criterion divides the primary carriers for imaging information, e.g., by its position inside the electromagnetic spectrum. Typical carriers are X-rays, light, sound, particle beams or magnetic resonance.

(2) *Spatial resolution:* The spatial resolution characterizes the differentiation of neighboring object points independent from the imaging contrast. This is also related to imaging accuracy. Its increase raises the amount of data tremendously.

(3) *Capability for stucture/tissue differentiation:* This evaluates the technique considering specific criteria for recognizing anatomic or functional objects, e.g., inner ear fluid, membranes, bone, vessels, and fibers. It is related to the imaging contrast and the process of (3D) image segmentation.

(4) *Surface vs. volume imaging:* Basically the imaging results may be divided into 2D and 3D surface imaging (picture/topography) and volume imaging (tomography).

(5) *Invasive vs. noninvasive:* The imaging procedure is classified 'invasive' in our terms if the geometry of the volume under investigation becomes affected. This is commonly the case in histologic sectioning or other techniques. In contrast it is declared 'noninvasive' if the investigation is carried out with specimens only for some few reasons (e.g., radiation biology), but preserves the complex morphology of the volume and its surrounding.

(6) *In vivo vs. in vitro:* Divides the techniques considering possible application in living humans, e.g., for diagnostic purposes.

During the study various physical approaches by theory and practice have been evaluated. Table 1 contains a selection and survey of those with special interest to inner ear imaging.

The data obtained by the various techniques, given in table 1, yield different kinds of representation depending on the application: morphometric data [11, 31–36], pictures (drawings, photographs) [12, 37–40], solid models [32, 41–48], or data-based geometry models [3, 49].

Several research activities deal with the simulation of sound transmission in the inner ear. Commonly those models are described by acoustic, electrical, or mechanical parameters. With the increasing performance of computers the numerically intensive Finite Element Method became more feasible. It requires two basic sets of parameters: (1) geometry properties (shapes, represented by surfaces or volumes) and (2) designation of localized material properties.

These include further parameters, e.g., coordinates of centers of gravity, Young's moduli, densities, and others. Often material properties should not be assumed homogeneous for single components. So far the geometry models used for Finite Element Analysis are designed using CAD software based on morphometric data, e.g., particular distance values. The main problem with them is the reproduction of the spatial relationship of the complex structures. Eventually, all these CAD models will always perform generalized views of biological structures, which usually show broad interindividual variations.

The inclusion of local variations returns the spatial resolution problem. Improving the resolution is in contrast to the increase of data amount related. Considering the assumptions of FE models, the tiniest structure inside the inner ear with high relevance to cochlear mechanics might be defined by the hair cells so far. That requires spatial resolution in the 1-μm range, neglecting the microstructural composition of the components under investigation. Concerning visualization and modeling applications, locally varying 'levels of detail' could be introduced.

This is due to the fact of huge data volumes to be processed. For 3D imaging, doubling of the resolution yields eight times of data points. A complete temporal bone specimen with intact middle and inner ear and removed outer ear canal may be assumed cube-shaped with edge distance of 20 mm. This distance is almost entirely occupied by the extents of the labyrinth. Furthermore supposed, the whole volume would be imaged by any technique at spatial resolution of 1 μm, and every voxel contains 8-bit data. This yields an 8-terabyte (10^{12}) data volume, which has to be processed and illustrates the extraordinary complexity of 3D data acquisition and processing of those actually microscopic structures.

Material and Methods

There are some particular conditions regarding temporal bone imaging. It contains the most solid bone of the human body. Therefore the highest concentration of calcium, or electron density, respectively, is found there. The geometrical dimensions of the anatomic structures of interest express high dynamics. They range from almost 20 mm (widest extent of the labyrinth) down to 1 μm (hair cell level). The entire hearing organ is located in a 8-cm^3 bone cube. Further dynamics is found in the target types: bone (surrounding the labyrinth and cochlea, the lamina spiralis ossea, or inside the modiolus), soft tissue (membranes, hair cells), and fluid-filled caves (bony/membranous labyrinth). The geometry of all these components affects the acoustic transfer behavior and thus should be taken into account.

This paper focuses on the introduction of microtomography into inner ear imaging. Microtomography was developed by the combination of direct magnification techniques with computed tomography principles. The physical carrier is provided by X-rays or synchrotron radiation. Furthermore, it may be divided into absorption and phase-contrast microtomography.

In contrast to clinical CT devices, X-ray micro-CT is equipped with microfocal spot tubes. Compared to synchrotron radiation they are permanently available, and cause low costs. But due to their broad-band radiation spectrum they show limitations regarding tissue differentiation, especially for soft tissues. Mainly bony and air-fluid-filled regions may be imaged with high contrast and resolutions <10 μm. Storage rings producing synchrotron radiation are situated on few locations worldwide only. Taking into account their imaging geometry, spatial resolution in the submicron range may be achieved. By using the coherence properties, chemical element-specific imaging becomes possible. Furthermore, the absorption microtomography can be turned to phase-contrast microtomography, which images the distribution of refractive indices and therefore will allow soft tissue differentiation [50]. Considering that physical background, the data revealed by the imaging process are not limited to geometry information, but contribute to the material parameter set as well (e.g., density distribution) and directly represent specific material inhomogeneities.

In this paper, results of imaging ethanol-fixated temporal bone specimens by absorption microtomography using both X-rays and synchrotron radiation are presented. The X-ray unit (Bundesanstalt für Materialprüfung, Berlin, Germany) [51] uses cone beam reconstruction technique and was set to tube voltage of 150 kV and current of 200 mA. It generated isotropic data sets with 60 μm (matrix 441 × 441 × 361) and 30 μm (831 × 831 × 729) spatial resolution. The tomographic sections provide sharp images with high contrast between bone and air or fluid respectively (fig. 1).

Generation of synchrotron radiation is a side effect in particle accelerators. It delivers a continuous spectrum from infrared to high-energy X-ray radiation. Because of the very low beam divergence, it

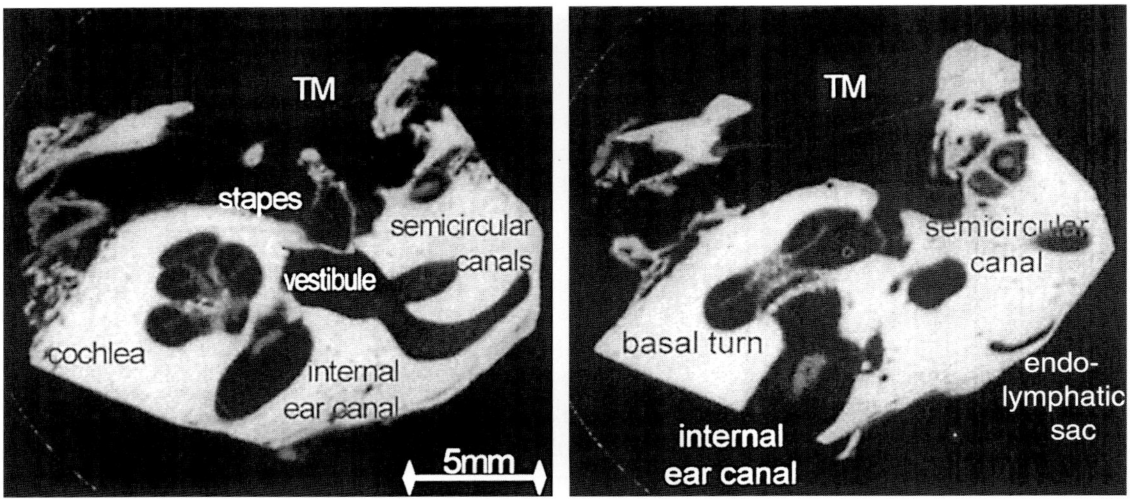

Fig. 1. X-ray microtomographic sections of temporal bone specimen, spatial resolution 30 μm.

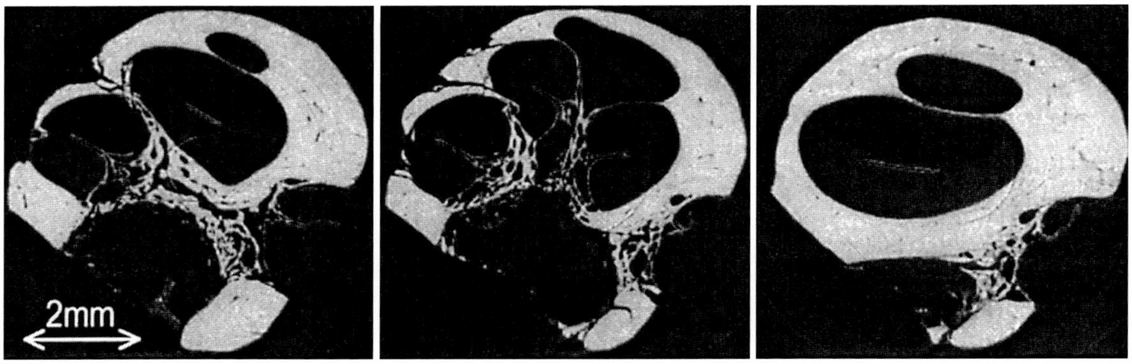

Fig. 2. Synchrotron radiation microtomographic sections of a cochlea specimen, spatial resolution 11 μm.

is used in parallel beam projection. A monochromator selects a specific wavelength suitable for the object under investigation. Nevertheless, intensity remains 10^4–10^6 times higher than with conventional X-ray tubes. Compared to them, synchrotron radiation provides some advantages: high intensity, collimation, tunable energy (5–50 KeV), and polarization. Typically it yields higher accuracy in the imaging quality [52]. Disadvantages are temporal and spatial beam stability, source availability, and limited probe dimensions due to the beam geometry.

Those experiments were performed at HASYLAB at DESY (Hamburg, Germany) in cooperation with physicists from the University of Dortmund (Germany). The radiation energy was 24 keV at 360 projections providing isotropic spatial resolution of about 11 μm (matrix 620 × 600 × 593). Due to the beam geometry, the specimen dimensions were limited. Therefore, a resected cochlea specimen underwent investigation (fig. 2).

Arranging all sections in a stack allows 3D reconstruction and segmentation. Segmentation provides the designation of individual colors to separate anatomic or functional objects for differentiation. This has been done using several 3D image-processing algorithms and software. All data processing and visualization was carried out using standard, but well-equipped personal computers (Pentium-II/266 MHz, 256 MB RAM, Windows 95, several peripherals).

Results

The processing of the raw tomographic data yielded a lot of different visualizations of the inner ear and internal temporal bone structures. The first pictures show the native spatial relation of the main components of the middle and inner ear. They were obtained by X-ray absorption microtomography (fig. 3).

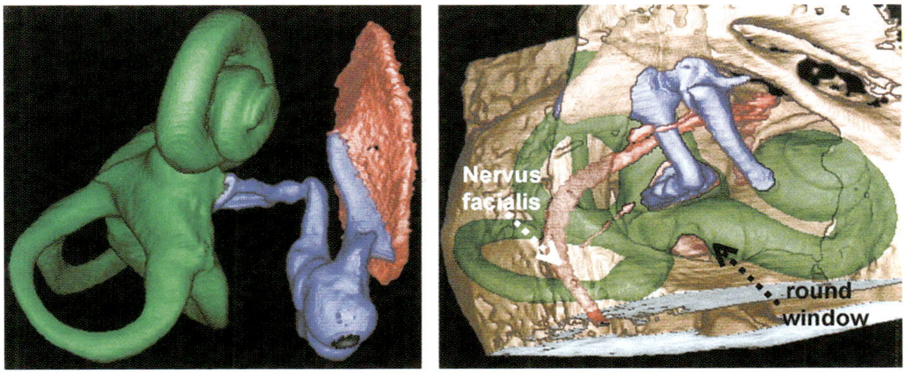

Fig. 3. X-ray absorption microtomography. Left: Segmentation of the fluid inside the bony labyrinth, ossicular chain and tympanic membrane in their native positions. Right: Location inside the temporal specimen.

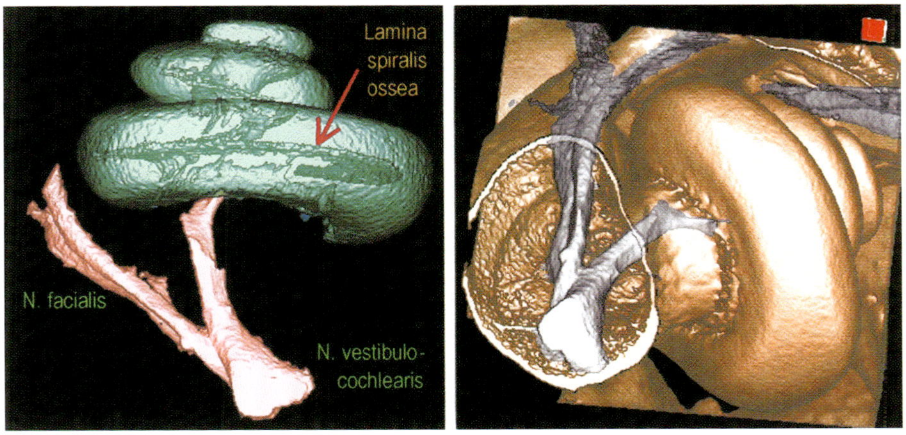

Fig. 4. X-ray absorption microtomography. Left: Segmentation of the cochlear fluid, lamina spiralis ossea, and nerves. Right: View inside the internal auditory meatus with course of the vestibulocochlear and facial nerves.

Due to their high contrast, imaging of the cochlear fluid and bony parts was possible. The very thin and hollow lamina spiralis ossea was imaged weakly, and the internal membranes not at all. Surprisingly the imaging of the course of several nerves succeeded, combined with views along the internal auditory meatus (fig. 4).

The introduction of synchrotron radiation into absorption microtomography has so far not improved the imaging results concerning soft tissues, but allowed higher spatial resolution. Again there is no indication for the basilar membrane or organ of Corti despite the spatial resolution in the 10-µm range. But some interest is directed onto the less bony section around the central diameter of the lamina spiralis ossea. Furthermore, small fractures caused during specimen preparation can be displayed very clearly (fig. 5, 6).

One of the goals of that study was to provide capabilities for geometry model derivation. Segmented objects may be transferrred from pixel into vector data by describing their surface. Now the data fit in CAD systems for adapting them to the simulation models. Another way is to determine relative coordinates of specific points along the segmented surfaces (fig. 7).

To fit into the processing performances of current computers and Finite Element Analysis systems and to ensure practical calculation times respectively, the high spatial resolution of the models has to be reduced. The model shown in figure 7 consists of 140,956 triangles defining its surface. There are several approaches to reduce that amount of elements to considerably lower levels by preserving the models' individuality. Figure 8 gives the same model reduced to 6,342 triangles.

Additionally the reconstructed volume data were visualized by means of animations and autostereoscopic displays. Furthermore, scaleable solid models have been produced by converting and putting the data into a rapid prototyping environment. They are hollow and may be filled with fluid for hydromechanical experiments. For exchanging the data, e.g., via the Internet, they have been transferred to VRML (virtual reality modeling language) models.

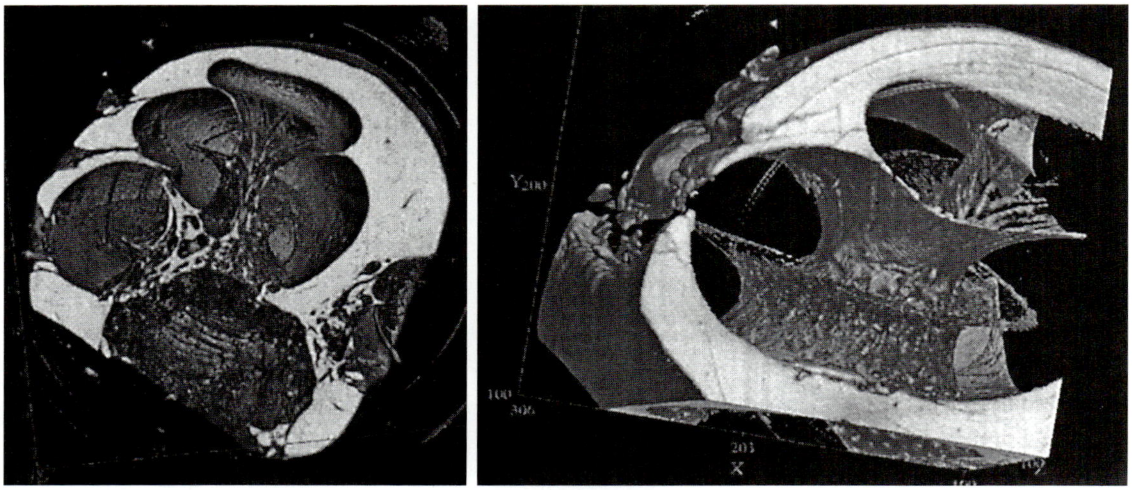

Fig. 5. Synchrotron radiation absorption microtomography. Left: Cut through the cochlea. Right: View onto modiolus and lamina spiralis ossea.

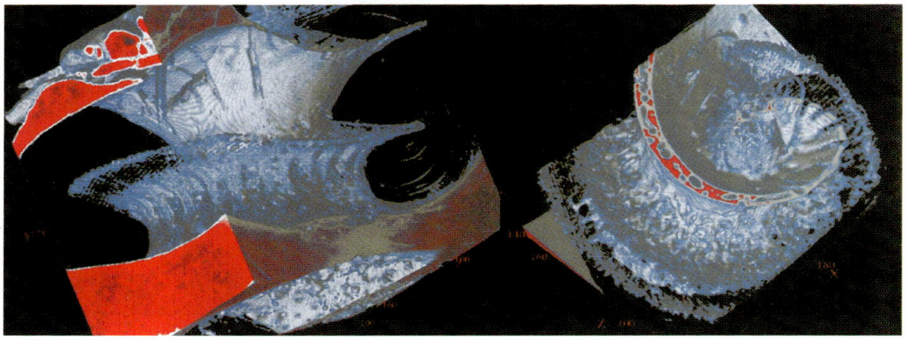

Fig. 6. Synchrotron radiation absorption microtomography. Left: Enlarged view onto modiolus and lamina spiralis ossea. Right: View onto the helicotrema region.

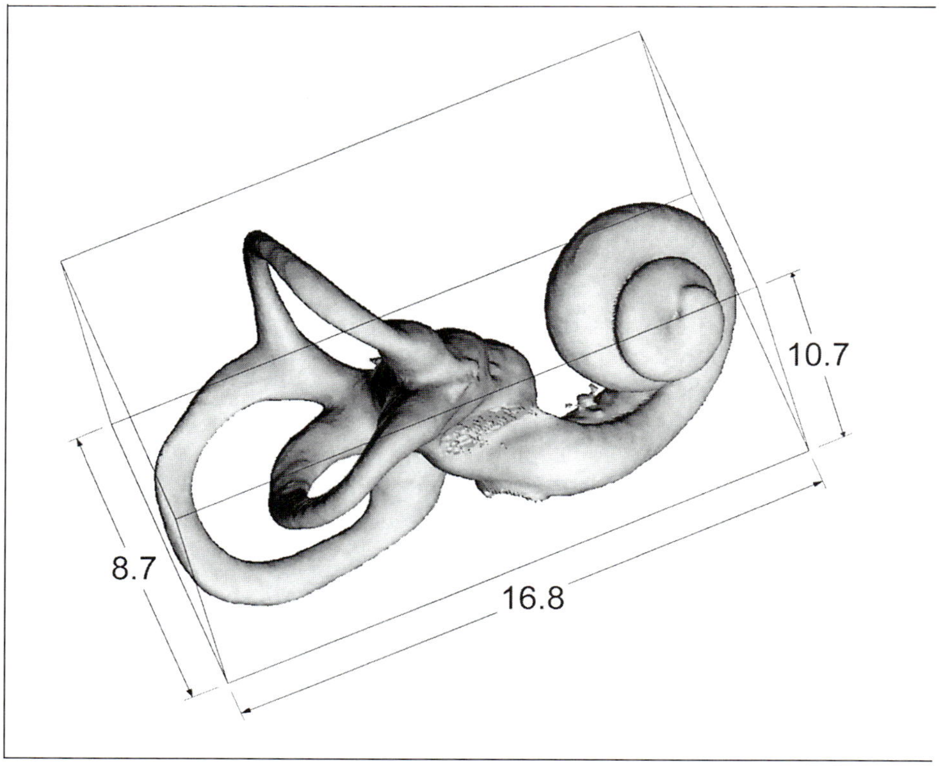

Fig. 7. Geometry modeling. Left: Extent of fluid inside the bony labyrinth. Right: Coordinate derivation for the same model (values in mm).

Conclusions

This paper presented a new approach for high-resolution, 3D imaging of the human inner ear and the hearing organ. It provides data and visualizations with spatial resolution in the 10-μm range. But, so far, some limitations remain unsolved, and new ones have appeared. Microtomography generally allows 3D data acquisition at resolution even higher yet, but generates data sets exceeding the capabilities of current standard computer equipment. The procedure is basically noninvasive, more accurate and much less time-consuming than comparable reconstructions from histologic sections. That opens opportunities for deriving interindividual models.

Absorption microtomography does not seem capable of imaging soft tissue components of the inner ear. For that purpose, phase-contrast microtomography is under evaluation. Because of the high radiation dose, that technique is not applicable for in vivo investigations of the inner ear up to now. Therefore, new approaches based on advanced incorporation of clinical CT equipment are under development [14].

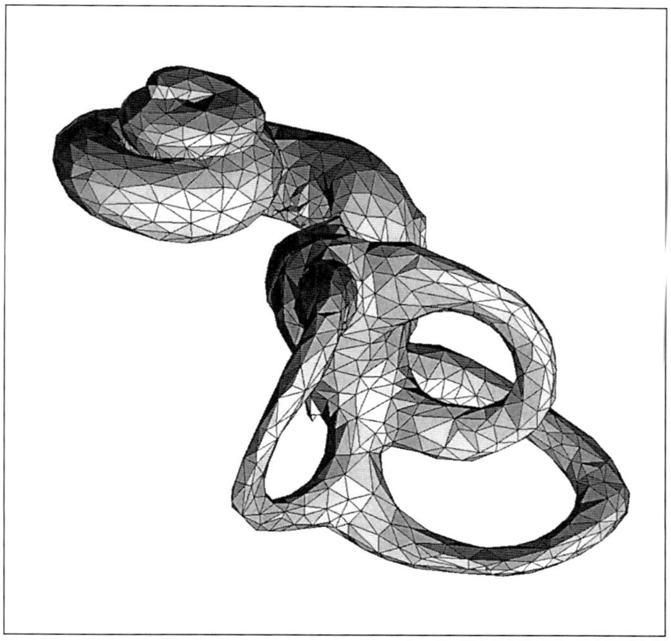

Fig. 8. Geometry modeling: model from figure 7 with reduced amount of elements (6,342 triangles).

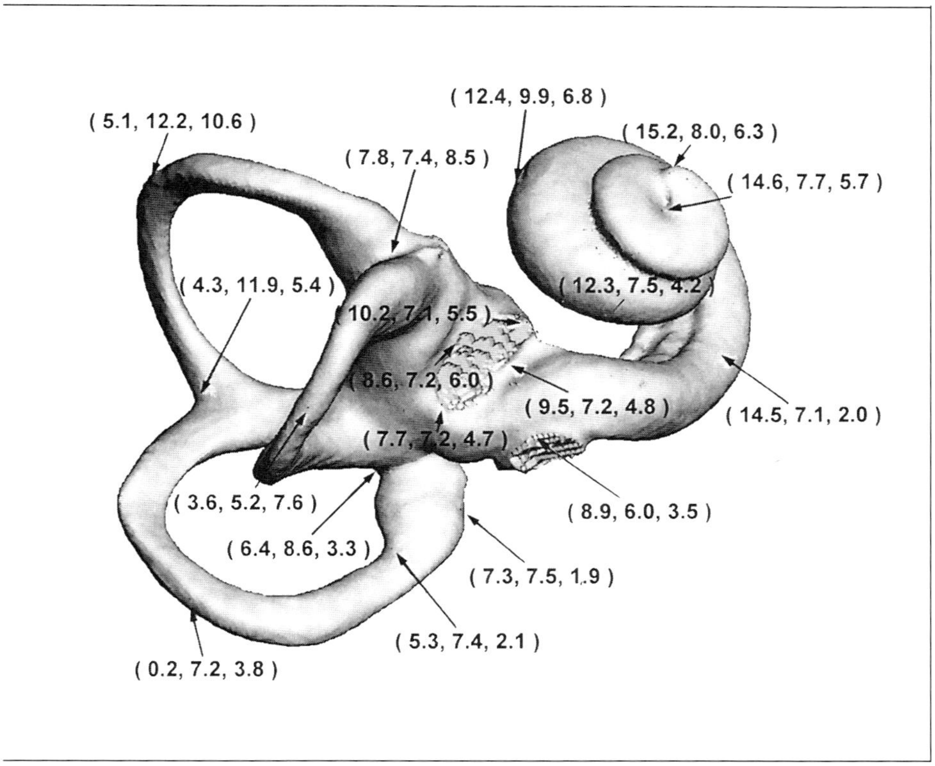

Acknowledgements

This work was motivated and supported by my former colleagues from the Department of Oto-Rhino-Laryngology of the University Hospital of the Dresden University of Technology, especially Dr. T. Zahnert, Prof. G. Hofmann and Prof. K.-B. Hüttenbrink. Cooperation is gratefully acknowledged to Dr. J. Goebbels at Bundesanstalt für Materialprüfung Berlin, and Dr. F. Beckmann and Prof. U. Bonse at HASYLAB at DESY Hamburg and Department of Physics/University of Dortmund.

References

1 Steele C: Comparison of 3-D mechanical models and measurement in the cochlea; in Biomechanics of Hearing. EUROMECH 368, Stuttgart, Sept 10–12, 1997, p 46.
2 Wilson JL, Henson MM, Gewalt SL, Keating AW, Henson OW: Reconstructions and cross-sectional area measurements from magnetic resonance microscopic images of the cochlea. Am J Otol 1996;17:347–353.
3 Stejskal V, Navara M, Ruzicka P: The modelling of inner ear acoustics using FEM; in Biomechanics of Hearing. EUROMECH 368, Stuttgart, Sept 10–12, 1997.
4 Ketten DR, Skinner MW, Wang G, Vannier MW, Gates GA, Neely JG: In vivo measures of cochlear length and insertion depth of nucleus cochlear implant electrode arrays. Ann Otol Rhinol Laryngol 1998;107:1–16.
5 Sapozhnikov A: Computer modelling of the implanted cochlea; thesis, Melbourne 1990.
6 Richter B, Jaekel K, Aschendorff A, Laszig R: Intracochleäre Position eines modiolusnahen CI-Elektrodenträgers bei Implantation und Explanation – eine Durchleuchtungsstudie. Poster Deutscher HNO-Kongress 1998, Hannover, 1998.
7 Phelps PD, Lloyd GAS: Radiology of the Ear. Oxford, Blackwell Scientific, 1983.
8 Zonneveld FW: Computed Tomography of the Temporal Bone and Orbit. München, Urban & Schwarzenberg, 1987.
9 Yamamoto E, Mizukami C, Isono M, Ohmura M, Hirono Y: Observation of the external aperture of the vestibulare aqueduct using three-dimensional surface reconstruction imaging. Laryngoscope 1991;101:480–483.
10 Takahashi H, Sando I: Computer-aided 3-D temporal bone anatomy for cochlear implant surgery. Laryngoscope 1990;100:417–421.
11 Skinner MW, Ketten DR, Vannier MW, Gates GA, Yoffie RL, Kalender WA: Determination of the position of nucleus cochlear implant electrodes in the inner ear. Am J Otol 1994;15:644–651.
12 Frankenthaler R, Moharir VM, Kikinis R, Kipshagen PV, Jolesz FA, Umans C, Fried MP: Virtual otoscopy. Otolaryngol Clin North Am 1998;31:383–391.
13 Reisser C, Schubert O, Forsting M, Sartor K: Anatomy of the temporal bone: detailed three-dimensional display based on image data from high-resolution helical CT: A preliminary report. Am J Otol 1996;17:473–479.
14 Vogel U, Schmitt T: 3D Visualization of Middle Ear Structures. Proc SPIE (Medical Imaging 1998), 1998, pp 141–151.
15 Vogel U, Hofmann G, Zahnert T, Hüttenbrink KB: Hochauflösend dreidimensionale Abbildung des menschlichen Innenohres und Ableitung eines skalierbaren körperlichen Modells; in Voigtmann L, Geyer P (eds): Tagungsband der 29. Jahrestagung der Dt Ges für Medizinische Physik, 1998, pp 373–374.
16 Brown CS, Burns DH, Spelman FA, Nelson AC: Computed tomography from optical projections for three-dimensional reconstruction of thick objects. Appl Opt 1992;31:6247–6254.
17 Voie AH, Spelman FA: Three-dimensional reconstruction of the cochlea from two-dimensional images of optical sections. Comput Med Imag Graph 1995;19:377–384.
18 Ghanem TA, Rabbitt RD, Tresco PA: Three-dimensional reconstruction of the membranous vestibular labyrinth in the toadfish, *Opsanus tau.* Hear Res 1998;124:27–43.
19 Reiss G: Electron microscopy in medicine and biology. http://www.stud.unihannover.de/user/77370/
20 Brogan M, Chakeres DW, Schmalbrock P: High-resolution 3DFT MR imaging of the endolymphatic duct and soft tissues of the otic capsule. Am J Neuroradiol 1991;12:1–11.
21 Denk W, Keolian RM, Ogawa S, Jelinski LW: Oscillatory flow in the cochlea visualized by a magnetic resonance imaging technique. Proc Natl Acad Sci USA 1993;90:1595–1598.
22 Leuwer R, Schubert R, Siepmann G: Die 3D-Darstellung hochauflösender MR-Tomographien des Innenohres. Laryngorhinootologie 1993;72:288–290.
23 Kumakawa K, Takemori S: High-resolution MR imaging of the inner ear. Acta Otolaryngol (Stockh) 1989(suppl 468):391–397.
24 Henson MM, Henson OW, Gewalt SL, Wilson JL, Johnson GA: Imaging the cochlea by magnetic resonance microscopy. Hear Res 1994;75:75–80.
25 Antunez JM, Galey FR, Linthicum FH, McCann GD: Computer-aided and graphic reconstruction of the human endolymphatic duct and sac. Ann Otol Rhinol Laryngol 1980;89:23–32.
26 Bagger-Sjöbäck D, Jansson B, Friberg U, Andersen HR: Three-dimensional anatomy of the human endolymphatic sac. Arch Otolaryngol Head Neck Surg 1990;116:345–349.
27 Lau S, Linthicum FH: Apparent apical endolymphatic hydrops – computer-aided three-dimensional reconstruction and histologic study of the apical turn of the cochlear duct. Am J Otol 1993;14:79–81.
28 Takagi A, Sando I: Computer-aided three-dimensional reconstruction: A method of measuring temporal bone structures including the length of the cochlea. Ann Otol Rhinol Laryngol 1989;98:515–522.
29 Green JD, Marion MS, Ericksson BJ, Robb RA, Hinojosa R: Three-dimensional reconstruction of the temporal bone. Laryngoscope 1990;100:1–4.
30 Bergmann K: Ein Computermodell des Innenohres. http://www.hu-berlin.de/inside/rz/mstat/avs/iohr.html
31 Curthoys IS, Markham CH, Curthoys EJ: Semicircular duct and ampulla dimensions in cat, guinea pig and man. J Morphol 1977;151:17–34.
32 Beck C, Bader J: Ein Beitrag zur feineren Anatomie des menschlichen Innenohres. Zusammengefasst dargestellt in einem neuen Labyrinthmodell. Arch Ohren Nasen Kehlkopfheilkd 1963;181:245–267.
33 Papangelou L: Volumetric study of the human internal auditory canal. J Laryngol 1974;88:349.
34 Sato H, Sando I, Takahashi H: Sexual dimorphism and development of the human cochlea. Computer 3-D measurement. Acta Otolaryngol (Stockh) 1991;111:1037–1040.
35 Santos MP: A computer-assisted morphometric method for 3-dimensional morphological reconstruction of the cochlea; thesis, Washington/Seattle 1987.
36 Linthicum FH, Galey FR: Computer-aided reconstruction of the endolymphatic sac. Acta Otolaryngol (Stockh) 1981;91:423–429.
37 Anson BJ, Donaldson JA: Surgical Anatomy of the Temporal Bone. New York, Raven Press, 1992.
38 Lang J: Klinische Anatomie des Ohres. Berlin, Springer, 1992.
39 Inside the Cochlea. http://www.boystown.org/cel/inside.htm
40 Harada T, Ishi S, Tayama N, Sugasawa M: Computer-aided three-dimensional reconstruction of the osseus and membraneous labyrinths. Eur Arch Otorhinolaryngol 1990;247:348–351.
41 Bader J: Ein neues Modell des menschlichen Labyrinths; Diss, Freiburg 1963.

42 Grant B: Virtual imaging helps surgeons navigate the temporal bone. Biophoton Int 1997 (Sept/Oct):19–20.
43 Tonndorf J: Fluid motion in cochlear models. J Acoust Soc Am 1957;29:558–568.
44 Bekesy GV: Experiments in Hearing. Huntington/NY, Krieger, 1960/1980.
45 Cannell JK: Cochlear models; thesis, Coventry 1969.
46 Helle R: Enlarged hydromechanical cochlea model with basilar membrane and tectorial membrane; in Zwicker E, Terhardt E (eds): Facts and Models in Hearing. New York, Springer, 1974, pp 77–85.
47 Chadwick RS, Adler D: Experimental observations of a mechanical cochlear model. J Acoust Soc Am 1975;58:706–710.
48 Zhou G, Bintz L, Anderson DZ: A life-sized physical model of the human cochlea with optical holographic readout. J Acoust Soc Am 1993;93:1516–1523.
49 Böhnke F, Arnold W: Biomechanisches 3D-FE Modell der Cochlea des Menschen. Biomed Tech 1998;43(suppl 1):26–27.
50 Bonse U, Beckmann F, Busch F, Günnewig O: X-ray microtomography using interferometric phase-contrast; in Thieme J, Schmahl E, Umbach E, Rudolph D (eds): X-Ray Microscopy and Spectromicroscopy. Heidelberg, Springer, 1996.
51 Riesemeier H, Goebbels J, Illerhaus B, Onel Y, Reimers P: 3-D Microcomputertomograph für die Werkstoffentwicklung und Bauteilprüfung. Deutsche Gesellschaft für Zerstörungsfreie Prüfung eV/Jubiläumstagung 60 Jahre DGZfP, Garmisch-Partenkirchen, 17–19 Mai 1993, pp 280–285.
52 Bonse U, Busch F: X-ray computed microtomography (μCT) using synchrotron radiation (SR). Prog Biophys Mol Biol 1996;65:133–169.

ORL

ORL 1999;61:268–274

Observations on Simultaneous Perilymphatic Motions and Cochlear Microphonics Suppression

E.-J. Haberland[a] H.J. Neumann[b]

[a]Klinik und Poliklinik für Hals-, Nasen-, Ohrenkrankheiten, Gesichts- und Halschirurgie, Martin-Luther-Universität Halle-Wittenberg, und [b]Klinik für Hals-Nasen-Ohrenheilkunde, Kopf- und Halschirurgie, Städtisches Klinikum 'Martha-Maria', Halle (Saale), Deutschland

Key Words

Cochlear mechanics · Basilar membrane · Perilymphatic pressure · Perilymphatic motion · Cochlear potentials · CM suppression · Tensor tympani muscle

Abstract

Very low frequencies interfere in the intact cochlea with higher frequencies and suppress these depending on the vibration phase of the low-frequency sound. Physiological functions of the body, mediated, for example, by the eardrum or perilymph coupling with the cerebrospinal fluid, cause a low-frequency pressure modulation of the perilymph, which generates a synchronous perilymphatic motion resulting from the unevenly distributed compliances in the cochlea. This slow streaming causes a displacement of the entire basilar membrane, with as a consequence a postponement of the operating point of the mechanoelectrical transducer as a result of the pressure drop in the helicotrema and the narrow apical cochlear turn. In this contribution, interference phenomena are described, which are caused by spontaneous contractions of the tensor tympani muscle and by respiration-synchronous perilymphatic flow. These two test signals have trapezoidal and triangular impulse functions. In both cases, as suppression pattern of the cochlear microphonics level-time function, the second derivative of the pressure-time function was observed. The suppression is found to lie between 1 and 2 dB. It depends on the level of the suppressed sound and shows a compressive nonlinearity.

Introduction

The hydrodynamics of the perilymph with regard to its importance for frequency selection has been widely examined. The biophysical aspects of the effects of convective transportation of the perilymph on kinetics of the metabolism are less well known. Such experiments require measurements of the stationary perilymphatic pressure and perilymphatic pressure dynamics at frequencies below the hearing range. Such measurements were carried out for example by Carlborg and co-workers [1, 2] from various clinical points of view. Our examinations on the guinea pig with the aim of a quantitative and qualitative description of perilymphatic pressure homeostasis were published in 1998 [3]. For these experiments, holes were drilled into the bone capsule of the cochlea for the posi-

KARGER

Fax + 41 61 306 12 34
E-Mail karger@karger.ch
www.karger.com

© 1999 S. Karger AG, Basel
0301–1569/99/0615–0268$17.50/0

Accessible online at:
http://BioMedNet.com/karger

Priv.-Doz. Dr. E.-J. Haberland
Univ.-HNO-Klinik, Magdeburger Strasse 12
D–06097 Halle (Saale) (Germany)
Tel. +49 345 557 1642, Fax +49 345 557 1859
E-Mail ernst.haberland@medizin.uni-halle.de

tioning of capillaries for pressure measurement and perilymphatic perfusion. The cochlear microphonics (CM) of the basal turn of the cochlea were recorded for the purpose of controlling the normal functioning of the cochlea. The perilymphatic system was acted on by transient, triangular, sinusoidal and trapezoidal volume impulses as test signals. As a consequence of the streamings caused thereby, a modulation of the CM could be determined. A similar modulation occurs as a result of perilymphatic motions which are evoked by body functions, as for example spontaneous contractions of the tensor tympani muscle (TTM) and respiration-synchronous pressure fluctuations of the cerebrospinal fluid (CSF) via the cochlear aqueduct. These influences work mostly in a disturbing manner, so that one cuts or cauterizes the tendon of the TTM [4] or, even during measurement, switches off the respirator. In this work, the type of CM modulation was studied from the point of view of both these streamings in a guinea pig model. Very low-frequency sounds at the eardrum generate comparable streamings in the perilymph.

Zwicker [5] examined the phenomenon of sound suppression in the normal speech range with deep sounds in the low hearing range using psychoacoustic methods on human beings. He explained this suppression as cochlear-mechanical. Other authors have discussed the phenomenon of basilar membrane movement resulting from animal experiments with the Mössbauer technique [6], capacitive probe [7] and AEP technique [8]. Among these are examinations involving measurement of the mechano-electrical transfer function between the auditory canal and the potential measurement electrode [9–11]. The pressure measurements in both perilymphatic scales by Franke and Dancer [12] and later by Décory et al. [10] complement the data.

Materials and Methods

Animals and Narcosis

The observations were carried out on adult female guinea pig (n = 3) with an average weight of 320 g each. Ketamine combination narcosis was applied (premedication: atropine sulfate 0.1 mg + Faustan 3.0 mg s.c. or i.m., 10 min; general anesthesia: Ketanest 20 mg i.m. or i.p., 5 min; local anesthesia: Xylocitin 0.5–1% 2–3 × s.c., 5 min later; the dissection then begins). Further injections during the experiments. Under this narcosis, spontaneous respiration and reflex activity remain in the oropharyngeal region.

Pressure Measurement

For positioning the glass capillary used for pressure measurement, the bulla tympanica was opened and at a 3-mm distance from the oval window a hole for the capillary was drilled. The bulla tympanica remained open during the measurements. The pressure transducer was connected with the capillary by means of a hose, which was filled with artificial perilymph. By means of electromechanical pressurizing of a connecting hose, an incremental 42-nl volume of artificial perilymph was injected through the capillary into the scala vestibuli and aspirated. This system, but filled with air, was also used for measuring the changes in pressure in the sealed-off auditory canal. Contractions of the TTM pull the eardrum inward and generate a hypotension impulse. These measurements could not be carried out during tone stimulation.

CM Registration

For CM registration a glass capillary with silver wire was placed into a second hole in the scala tympani, approximately 3.5 mm from the round window. Only the tip was immersed in the perilymph. Both capillaries were fixed with acrylic glue. This single electrode technology is suitable for stable monitoring of CM over a number of hours. It delivers the vector sum of CM for a considerable part of the first cochlear turn.

Tone Stimulation

Stimulation of the animals with sinusoidal tones was brought about within a closed system. Because of the open bulla, ambient noise at 48 dB SPL affected the eardrum of the animal in the lab and generated a wide-band CM response. This CM level was used as benchmark for all further CM values.

Induced TTM Contraction Test Signal

Under the anesthesia described above, repeated spontaneous contractions of the TTM occur with the following parameters [3]: Frequency 30 min^{-1} SD ± 11.5 (n = 15, n is the number of animals considered), half value of width 363 ms SD ± 100 (n = 6), pressure amplitude in the perilymph 62 Pa SD ± 25 (n = 15). The time course has a trapezoidal character with a faster increase than decrease. The spectral components with the highest energy extend as high as 2.3 Hz, higher frequencies being damped by 40 dB.

Respiration-Induced Test Signal

The cochlear aqueduct of the guinea pig is open in many cases. The measurable trapezoidal pressure fluctuations in the CSF propagate in this case directly into the perilympathic space. Because of low-pass filtering, caused by the compliance of the perilymphatic space and the resistance of the cochlear aqueduct, they have a triangular appearance there with approximately 20% of the magnitude of the TTM impulse. Further details on the method are to be found in Neumann and Haberland [3]. The care and use of the animals used in this study were carried out in accordance with the actual guidelines of the animal care committee.

Results

Spontaneous contractions of the TTM sometimes occur singly, sometimes at irregular intervals and sometimes even triggered by respiration. Figure 1a shows a typical example of the summation of the two dynamic influences on the perilymph pressure, TTM contraction and respiration. The onset of contraction begins at different phases of

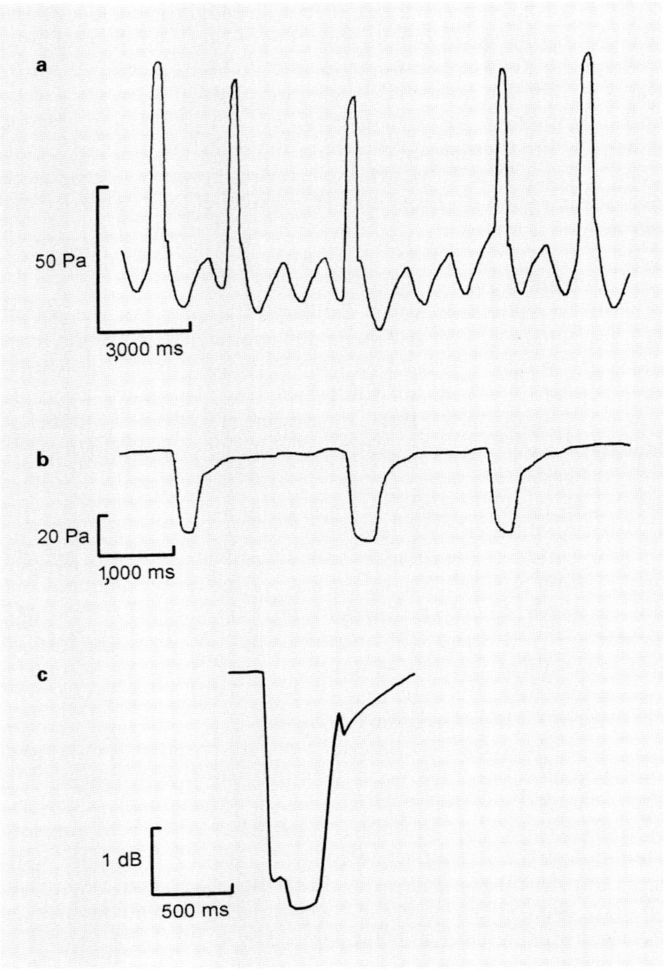

1

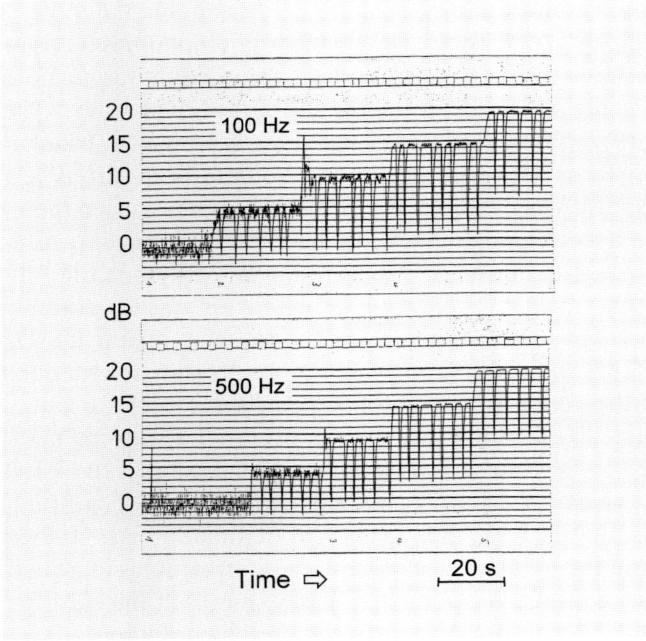

2

Fig. 1. a Spontaneous contractions of the TTM generate pulse-shaped pressure peaks in the perilymph, which add together to form the triangular pattern of the respiration effect. **b** The inward movement of the eardrum due to TTM contraction generates negative pressure impulses in the sealed auditory canal. **c** Suppression of the 10-dB CM level of a sinusoidal tone of 1,000 Hz due to contraction of the TTM.

Fig. 2. Influence of TTM contractions on different CM levels (re 20 μV), on stimulation with continuous sinusoidal tones of 100 and 500 Hz.

breathing in. The form of the peaks changes according to the superposition of triangular fluctuations in pressure due to respiratory factors. In order to get a better picture of the actual course of temporal movement of the eardrum, the time function of hypotension in the sealed auditory canal under TTM contraction was plotted (fig. 1b). This gives a qualitative picture of the eardrum movement. The magnitude of the resulting hypotension depends on the volume of the auditory canal, the measuring system and the opening of the bulla tympanica, and should therefore be considered as relative. Any return effect of perilymphatic pressure fluctuations by way of the ossicles on the eardrum should be neglected in this case. Figure 1c shows the suppression pattern of such a TTM pressure pulse. As a result of the increased tension of the TTM at 1,000 Hz tone stimulation, stiffening of the eardrum causes a change in impedance, which appears in the CM suppression pattern as a transfer loss of several dB. The two kinks at the drop and rise of the curve cannot be determined from the pressure response. They apparently result from nonlinearities in the cochlear mechanoelectrical transduction.

Figure 2 shows two examples of the dependence of suppression on the CM level registered. A linear behavior is only to be determined in the case of the first and second level steps. The baseline was determined on the basis of the CM level fluctuations due to ambient noise in the laboratory and biological disturbances at the electrode. There is a noticeable difference in summation of this broad-band noise at constant CM level of sound and at various frequencies. The maximum vibration of the basilar membrane (BM) lies at 500 Hz basally shifted, so that also the BM displacement and therefore the CM near the electrode is greater, given the same vibration amplitude at

3

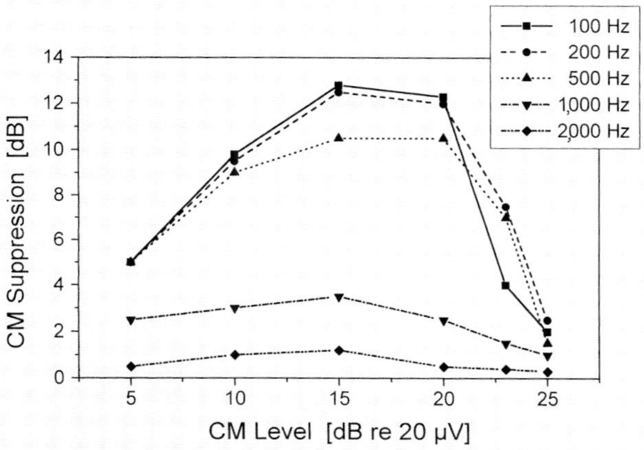

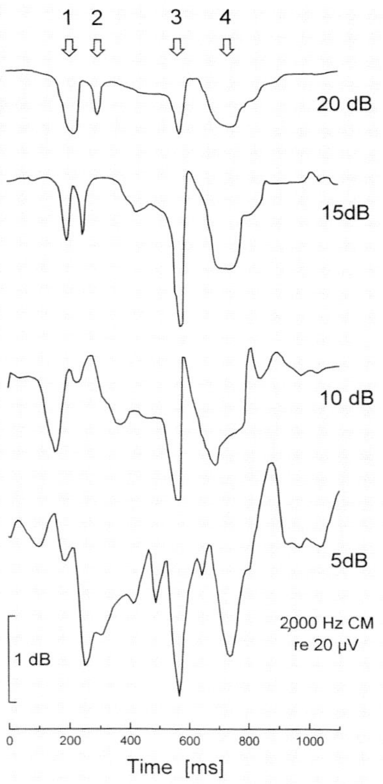

4

Fig. 3. Diminution of sinusoidal tone CM levels due to spontaneous contractions of the TTM in dependence on the CM level at 5 frequencies.

Fig. 4. Fine structure of the suppression pattern of a 2,000-Hz sinusoidal tone which was registered with 4 different contractions of the TTM. Each contraction has a different CM level. Arrows 1 and 2 mark the events of the contraction period, and arrows 3 and 4 the events of the relaxation.

the best frequency position. Further, the fact that there is an unknown spread of CM from all hair cells through the spatially distributed electric impedance of the cochlear tissue needs to be considered. The magnitude of the suppression at further frequencies and at a CM level of 25 dB is shown in figure 3. Between 100 and 2,000 Hz, the level dependence of the CM suppression is found to be in principle the same at all frequencies. From 15 dB CM level, the CM generator is increasingly saturated. From 20 dB the decreasing portion of the CM characteristic curve of the cochlea comes into play. The frequency dependence up to 1,000 Hz is a consequence of the properties of the eardrum. The change in eardrum impedance plays only a subordinate role from 2,000 Hz due to TTM contraction. This frequency is therefore especially well suited for examination of the influence of basilar membrane vibration caused by slow perilymphatic motions in the scala vestibuli (SV) and the scala tympani (ST).

The fine structure of the suppression pattern of a constant 2,000-Hz tone (fig. 4), produced by TTM contractions, becomes clear at higher levels, while as a CM level of 5 dB over ambient noise suppression peaks and troughs almost vanish under random fluctuations. The contraction and relaxation phases of the TTM are marked by two suppression peaks each. Most striking is peak 3, which marks the beginning of the relaxation. It was therefore also used as synchronization for the comparison of the four curves. Relaxation of the TTM means that pressure in the perilymph begins to decrease. The pressure outflow lies in the SV. As a consequence of hypotension, perilymph streams through the helicotrema and the narrow upper cochlear turn into the SV. This brings about a pressure difference between the scalae, which however owing to its spectral components below the hearing range leads to bending of the entire basilar membrane like a plate. This effect is caused by streaming dynamic considerations and could be explained by the different cross sections and different streaming speeds resulting from them. Change of the sign of the derivative leads between peak 3 and peak 4 in trace c to a slight increase in CM.

The aforementioned contraction rate of the TTM is only a mean value that in the individual case can be roughly as great as the respiration rhythm. Then there is a beat between the two periodic pressure influences on the

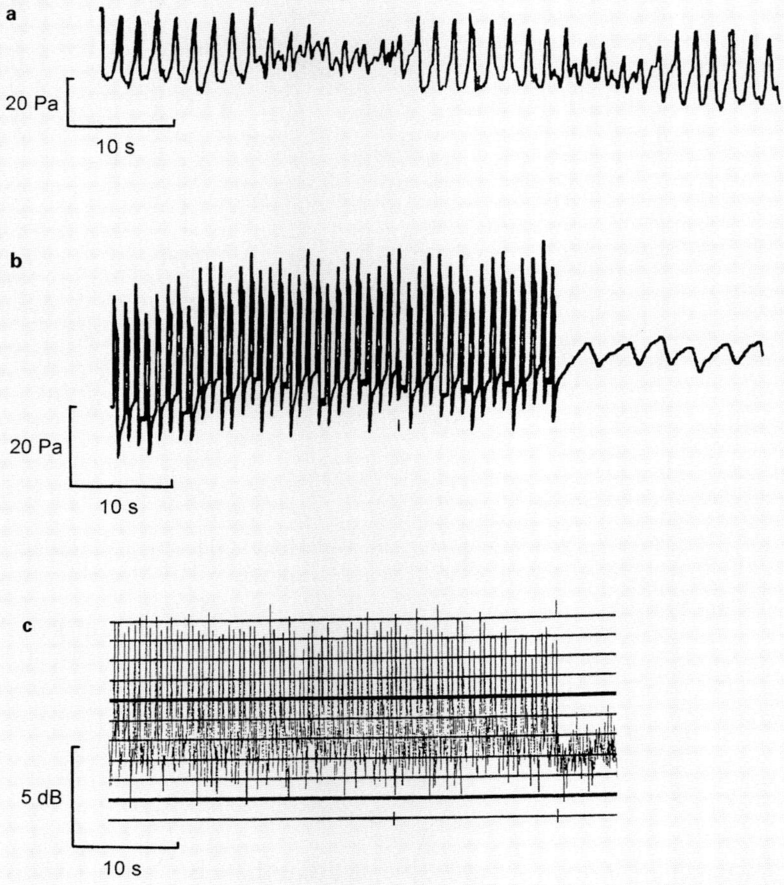

Fig. 5. **a** Beats of pressure impulses due to rhythmic contractions of the TTM and respiration-conditioned pressure fluctuations which have in this case approximately the same frequency in the perilymph of the scala vestibuli. **b** Superposition of respiration-conditioned pressure fluctuations and pressure impulses from incremental volumes (42 nl, 400 ms) artificially injected into the perilymphatic space and subsequently aspirated. The last 20 s are shown without incremental injection. **c** Simultaneously registered CM levels regarding trace **b**. The spikes are the sum of the responses of the CM of the impulse rise and decay as well as low-frequency vibration (65 Hz) artifacts of the electromechanical impulse production apparatus.

perilymph (fig. 5a) which has no zero-minimum because of the somewhat different amplitudes and forms. In trace b of figure 5 the respiration-conditioned streaming and incremental volumes, whose injection/aspirations rates amount to 3- to 4-fold the respiration frequency, are shown. On inflow and outflow they generate low-frequency CM (fig. 5c) which are still overlaid by CM from unavoidable oscillations of the volume stimulation system (65 Hz). These low-frequency CM are clearly modulated by the respiration-conditioned perilymph streaming. This effect is shown in figure 6. There are 12 respirations and 23 CM suppressions ('negative peaks'). Events with direction reversal are counted as peaks. The match is not very exact because the sampling rate with incremental volumes amounts to only the 3- to 4-fold the respiration frequency. In the middle of the curve, the agreement between direction reversal in the respiration-pressure characteristic and the occurrence of CM suppressions can easily be seen. This corresponds to the second derivative of the respiration-conditioned pressure-time curve with respect to time.

Discussion

The observations presented confirm amongst other things the well-known fact that for very low-frequency pressure modulation of the perilymph, the suppression pattern of CM corresponds to the second derivative of the pressure-time function. The suppression pattern shown in this work can be described in accordance with the model of Zwicker [5] (fig. 7). This model was used for the explanation of the results of psychoacoustic examinations. With clinical application of this knowledge it is normal to

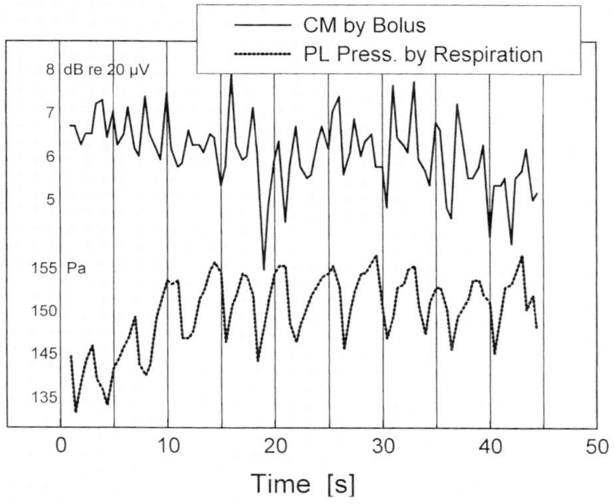

6

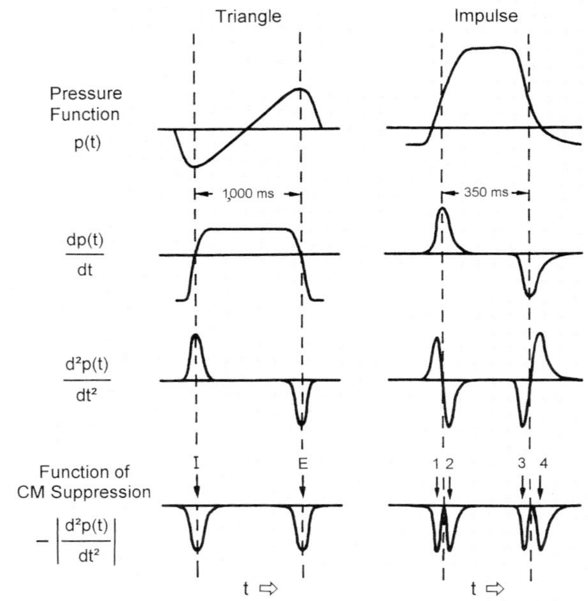

7

Fig. 6. Synchronous representation of the respiration-conditioned perilymph pressure fluctuations (bottom), calculated from figure 5 b, and fluctuations of the streaming-induced CM level evoked thereby (top), calculated from figure 5 c.

Fig. 7. Explanation of the CM suppressions shown in figures 4 and 6, both evoked by slow perilymphatic motion following Zwicker's model [5]. The time function of respiration-conditioned perilymphatic pressure fluctuations is approximately triangular and mostly it has a slower increase on inspiration (I) in comparison with expiration (E). Two suppression peaks originate with the negative absolute value of the second derivative of the pressure function. The pressure impulses due to TTM contraction are approximately rectangular with somewhat rounded contours. They generate four suppression peaks with the negative absolute value of the second derivative of the pressure function.

work with low-frequency sinusoidal suppressor tones of high intensity [13]. The phenomena examined in this work are caused by nonsinusoidal signals. Their spectra have their main components in the infrasound range. In comparison with audiofrequencies, they generate a clear streaming in perilymph. Approximately half the volume of the apical cochlear turn in the guinea pig is displaced with each contraction of the TTM. This perilymphatic motion has a possible significance for convective transport. This streaming generates a pressure loss in the helicotrema and in the narrow apical cochlear turn, which was determined by acoustic [9] as well as hydrodynamic methods [3]. Since the input impedance of the guinea pig BM and helicotrema at very low frequencies is purely resistive, the expected agreement of these values was confirmed. The pressure differences of a calculated magnitude up to 20 Pa caused by volume fluctuation in the helicotrema lead to the expectation of a noticeable displacement of the BM, which amounts to 0.4 nm at 0 dB SPL [7]. LePage [7] has measured the BM movement produced by artificial respiration (25 nm) and heartbeat (10 nm) in the paralyzed guinea pig by capacitive probe technique. The second pattern of perilymphatic motion examined was the respiration pattern. Pressure coupling occurs predominantly via the cochlear aqueduct. If surgically sealed, the measurable, respiration-conditioned pressure waves do not disappear completely but to a certain extent remain [3]. This is caused by dynamic pressure coupling to the respiration rhythm via the vascular bed of the epithelium in the scalae. This uneven distribution of compliances in the perilymphatic space also causes each volume demand to evoke streamings in the entire perilymph. The fluid from the cochlear aqueduct does not affect the vestibular side of the BM, but rather the ST side, unlike the flow from the base of stapes. It is therefore reasonable to expect that the greatest suppression should occur during the rise in pressure instead of its decrease. In figure 6 this can indeed be seen, but is not clearly demonstrated. A higher test impulse rate would improve the resolution.

The phenomena observed can be summarized as follows: (a) Contractions of the TTM and the respiration rhythm appear in the perilymph as rectangular and triangular pressure-time functions with pressure amplitudes of several tens of Pascal. (b) The unevenly distributed compliances in the perilymphatic space lead to streamings in the helicotrema with the consequence of a pressure difference between the scalae and thus to a displacement of the basilar membrane. (c) The suppression pattern of sinusoidal tones corresponds to the negative absolute value of the second derivative of the pressure-time function. (d) The clearest suppression originates with the onset of a pressure decrease in the scala vestibuli.

References

1 Carlborg B, Densert B, Densert O: Functional patency of the cochlear aqueduct. Ann Otol Rhinol Laryngol 1982;91:209–215.

2 Carlborg B, Farmer J: Transmission of cerebrospinal fluid pressure via the cochlear aqueduct and endolymphatic sac. Am J Otolaryngol 1983;4:273–282.

3 Neumann HJ, Haberland EJ: Biophysikalische Untersuchungen der Perilymphbewegung und Sauerstoffdiffusion im cochleären Perilymphraum unter pathophysiologischen Bedingungen. Eine tierexperimentelle Studie. Marburg, Tectum Verlag, 1998.

4 Dallos P, Cheatham MA, Ferraro J: Cochlear mechanics, nonlinearities, and cochlear potentials. J Acoust Soc Am 1974;55:597–605.

5 Zwicker E: Masking-period patterns produced by very low frequency maskers and their possible relation to basilar-membrane displacement. J Acoust Soc Am 1977;61:1031–1040.

6 Robles L, Ruggero M, Rich N: Mössbauer measurements of basilar membrane tuning curves in the chinchilla. J Acoust Soc Am 1985;76:155–159.

7 LePage E: The application of a capacitive probe technique for direct observation of electromechanical processes in the guinea pig cochlea. J Acoust Soc Am 1987;82:126–138.

8 Gerull G, Mrowinski D, Nubel K: Low-frequency masking of brainstem potentials. Scand Audiol 1991;20:227–234.

9 Dallos P: Low-frequency auditory characteristics: Species dependence. J Acoust Soc Am 1970;48:489–499.

10 Décory L, Franke RB, Dancer AL: Measurement of the middle ear transfer function in cat, chinchilla and guinea pig; in Dallos P, Matthews JW, Ruggero MA, Steele CR (eds): The Mechanics and Biophysics of Hearing. Berlin, Springer, 1990, pp 270–277.

11 Magnan P, Dancer A, Probst R, Smurczynski J, Avan P: Intracochlear acoustic pressure measurements. Transfer functions of the middle ear and cochlear mechanics. Audiol Neurootol 1999;4:123–128.

12 Franke R, Dancer A: Cochlear mechanisms at low frequencies in the guinea pig. Arch Otorhinolaryngol 1982;234:213–218.

13 Mrowinski D, Gerull G, Nubel K, Scholz G: Masking and pitch shift of tone bursts and clicks by low-frequency tones. Hear Res 1995;85:95–102.

ORL

ORL 1999;61:275–286

Nonlinear Mechanics of the Inner Ear and Its Relation to Otoacoustic Emissions: Two Steps on the Way to a Mathematical Model of DPOAE Generation

Michael Ganz[a] Michael F. Berg[b]

[a]Department of Experimental Audiology, University of Magdeburg,
[b]Audiological Laboratory, ENT University Hospital, Erlangen, Germany

Key Words

Inner ear · Otoacoustic emissions · Model calculations · Nonlinearity · Distortion product

Abstract

Among clinical users of the registration of distortion product otoacoustic emissions (DPOAE), the understanding of the basic causality and interpretation of the phenomenon is not yet widely spread, nor is the expected influence of the middle ear and ear canal clear. On the other side, the effort in mathematical modeling of middle and inner ear structures is driven very far by now. We are convinced, though, that the essentials of an effect as DPOAE generation must be understandable from quite simple models. In a *first step* de Boer's one-dimensional model was adopted and expanded by a weak frictional and a weak elastic nonlinearity, respectively. By means of perturbation theory the weakly nonlinear problem is converted in an approximation series of linear problems. So it is solvable by the common methods of linear differential equations (DEs), above all the superposition principle can be used. At the same time a structure of causality is introduced: Sources for outgoing waves are in first order approximation formed by incoming waves, and so they can be localized. The calculations show clearly that of all six cubic distortions only the $2f_1 - f_2$ term does have a source in its 'allowed' region and so can travel outward. We can use the calculated DPOAE to study the influence of middle ear, external ear canal and probe plug. Some problems remain: the weakly nonlinear model in first order does not give account for proper $L_{dp} = f(L_1, L_2)$ and $L_{dp} = f(f_2/f_1)$ dependency, nor does it deliver additional sources or the effect of additional suppressor tones. In a *second step*, therefore, we replace de Boer's simple model basilar membrane (BM) by a doubly resonant, coupled tectorial/basilar membrane (TM/BM) system. By feedback now we introduce a strong nonlinearity, which we can mathematically care for by an iterative feedback loop. The algorithm shapes the incoming waves according to strong compressive nonlinearity. More relastic incoming waves yield better source terms, and after optimization of the mistuning function between TM and BM the model now is able to deliver qualitatively correct L_{dp} (L_1,L_2) and $L_{dp}(f_2/f_1)$ dependencies.

Introduction

Numerous mathematical models have been used to reproduce the 'traveling wave' and the tonotopy of the cochlea [1, 3]. Only few attempts, however, have been made up to now to model the OAE generation mathemati-

KARGER

Fax + 41 61 306 12 34
E-Mail karger@karger.ch
www.karger.com

© 1999 S. Karger AG, Basel
0301–1569/99/0615–0275$17.50/0

Accessible online at:
http://BioMedNet.com/karger

Michael Ganz, Abteilung für Experimentelle Audiologie und Medizinische Physik
Otto-von-Guericke-Universität, Leipziger Strasse 44
D–39120 Magdeburg (Germany)
Tel. +49 391 6713882, Fax +49 391 6713888
E-Mail michael.ganz@medizin.uni-magdeburg.de

cally [4, 5]. The latter would be of some clinical relevance, nevertheless. The registration and interpretation of TOAEs and DPOAEs are daily routine in audiological practice, whilst a real understanding of the generation of OAEs and the possible causes of pathological deviations is still missing. So for example the question still stands, whether OAE generation needs real active motility or if slowly adjustable nonlinearity alone is sufficient.

The aim of this ongoing study is: (a) to model DPOAE generation mathematically; (b) to study the influence of middle ear and ear canal on the registration of DPOAE; (c) to adapt the model so as to produce a substantially correct $L_{dp} = f(L_1,L_2)$ dependency; (d) to adapt the model so as to produce a basically correct $L_{dp} = f(\omega_2/\omega_1)$ dependency; (e) eventually to adapt the model to show correctly the effect of suppressor tones, and (f) later on to study the generation of the fluctuating fine structure of the DPOAE.

It turned out very soon that an approach in several steps was necessary, of which the first two are to be reported here.

Step 1: Weak Nonlinearity in a 1-D Model

Using de Boer's 1-D model [1] and introducing a cubic perturbation term, we produced our first model DPOAEs [4, 5].

Methods

We have found a realistic way to model the generation of the cubic difference tone, frequency $2\omega_1 - \omega_2$, as commonly measured in DPOAE registration [5]. Because we thought DP generation a very fundamental process, not too sensitive to fine details of the cochlea model, we had adapted the simple one-dimensional cochlea model published by de Boer [1]. We start from inertia and incompressibility of the inner ear fluids and inertia, friction and elasticity of the basilar membrane (BM). Then we set up the model as three coupled differential equations (DEs), which describe the interdependencies of local pressure p(x,t), alternating longitudinal lymph velocity u(x,t), and the transverse velocity of the cochlear partition v(x,t) functions. (We designate distance from stapes by x, time by t. For more details, see Appendix 1.) For the pressure and BM velocity function we have one DE

$$Z_0 v(x,t) + 2\,p(x,t) = 0 \qquad (1)$$

Here Z_0 is a linear differential operator, in the simple case of de Boer's model

$$Z_0 v(x,t) = M \cdot \frac{d}{dt} v(x,t) + R(x) \cdot v(x,t) + C(x) \cdot \int v(x,t)dt$$

Here the M, R, and C are mass, friction and stiffness per unit area. We are not bound to this form. Any linear differential operator in t will do. We shall have reasons later to use a more complicated form of Z_0.

The linear DE (1) together with the two additional DEs from de Boer's model, describing inertia and incompressibility of lymph flow, can be solved sequentially to deliver first p(x,t), then u(x,t) and v(x,t), exhibiting realistic BM-traveling waves with correct tonotopy. We have expanded the Z_0 by an additional nonlinear, cubic term Z_1, which can be of several forms

e.g.: $Z_1\, v(x,t) = R\, v^3(x,t)$	miming a nonlinear friction or
e.g.: $Z_1\, v(x,t) = C\, (\int v(x,t)dt)^3$	giving a nonlinear elasticity.

Other types of 'perturbation' of the linear equation are possible of course. The complete equation can then be rewritten to:

$$Z_0\, v(x,t) + 2\, p(x,t) = -\varepsilon\, Z_1\, v(x,t)$$

The size of the additional term is made adjustable by a so-called perturbation parameter ε. If ε is put to zero, we have the 'unperturbed' problem: a linear one. When ε is non-zero, the DE is more or less nonlinear and all the common solution methods, including the superposition principle, cannot be used any longer.

According to H. Poincaré, a small perturbation will have only small effects on the solutions p(x,t) and v(x,t), meaning that it makes sense to try a power series expansion of the solutions of the form

$$v(x,t) = v_0(x,t) + \varepsilon\, v_1(x,t) + \varepsilon^2\, v_2(x,t) + \ldots$$
$$p(x,t) = p_0(x,t) + \varepsilon\, p_1(x,t) + \varepsilon^2\, p_2(x,t) + \ldots$$

Insertion of these series into the DE and sorting out the equations by powers of ε gives a series of linear DEs, namely:

unperturbed	$Z_0 v_0 + 2p_0 = 0$
in 1st order	$Z_0 v_1 + 2p_1 = -Z_1(v_0^3)$
in 2nd order	$Z_0 v_2 + 2p_2 = -Z_1(3v_0^2 v_1)$
in 3rd order	$Z_0 v_3 + 2p_3 = -Z_1(3v_0 v_1^2 + 3v_0^2 v_2)$
in 4th order	$Z_0 v_4 + 2p_4 = -Z_1(3v_0^2 v_3 + 6v_0 v_1 v_2 + v_1^3)$

The relatively simple problem now is to solve these DEs step by step. All of them are linear and the homogeneous part is the same for all. Besides, a kind of *causality* is introduced. The solution v_0 of the unperturbed DE gives the right-hand side (RHS) of the inhomogenous DE, and so can be interpreted as *the source* of the first order solution.

The solutions of the first two DEs give the source term for the second order perturbed DE and so on. So the DE system is solvable and actually the first order perturbed DE already delivers the most important phenomenon: the distortion product and the place of its generator around the characteristic site for f_2.

Even the correct size of the distortion product can be generated by proper choice of ε, as long as the problem is only weakly nonlinear, i.e. the necessary ε is small in some sense. It turns out that a solution in space and time cannot be acquired but by transformation of the DEs and functions into the frequency domain. (For details, see Appendices 1 and 2.)

Results

The first step investigations and results have been reported in more detail elsewhere [4, 6]. Therefore we shall give only a concise account here. Using the model parameter set of table 1, we solved the DE for $p_\omega(x)$ in several frequencies. Disregarding certain constant factors,

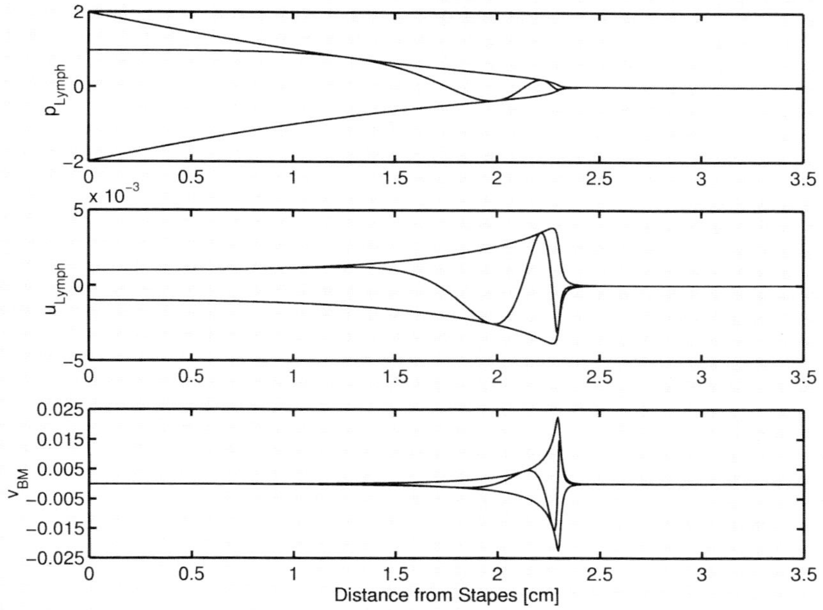

Fig. 1. It is quite common to show only the typical peak-shaped elongation or velocity functions of the cochlear partition when the inner ear is fed by a harmonic. It is remarkable that $|p_\omega(x)|$ does decrease in a monotonous way from the stapes to the cut-off site, and that $|u_\omega(x)|$, the longitudinal component of the lymph movement, is more or less constant up to the same place. (The peak amplitude of the traveling wave for input levels of 60 dB is about 1 nm, which still is about a factor of 1 million times smaller than the diameter of the scales. It must be stressed therefore that while the x-axis in this diagram is enlarged by a factor of about 2, the vertical axis enlarged by a factor of 20 millions!)

the first and second derivative with respect to x then deliver $u_\omega(x)$ and $v_\omega(x)$. On a computer screen it is easy then to display animated traveling waves and to interactively test out the influence of the model parameters on tonotopy and shape of the wave functions. [Contact the authors by E-Mail for binaries or Pascal sources of their programs.] For print we must confine to snapshots like figure 1, showing the waves and their envelopes for a frequency of 200 Hz. After this zero order calculation the sources of DPOAE in first order perturbation can be formed from the zero order $v_{\omega_1}(x)$ and $v_{\omega_2}(x)$ functions, the 'incoming waves'. There are six different source terms according to the six different cubic distortion frequency components (details in Appendix 2). The only source situated in an 'allowed' region, i.e. laying basically of its characteristic surging place, where traveling waves can be generated, is the one belonging to $2\omega_1 - \omega_2$. It is proportional to $v^2_{\omega_1}(x)\cdot v^*_{\omega_2}(x)$. The product vanishes where $v_{\omega_2}(x)$ falls to zero and therefore the first order source is located 'below' $|v_{\omega_2}(x)|$. In fact, the source term has a sharp peak just at the surging site of ω_2 and a kind of short basal tail, both having a slightly ocmplicated phase. (In fact it does not have much similarity to the intersection triangle shown by some authors.) This source generates two traveling waves at the same time: (1) a wave traveling towards the apex –

Table 1. Model parameters of the weak nonlinear model (step 1)

Parameter		
C(x)	$1.58\cdot10^9\cdot e^{-\alpha x}$	$\frac{dyn}{cm^3}$
M	0.1	$\frac{g}{cm^2}$
R(x)	$\delta\sqrt{CM}$	$\frac{dyn\cdot s}{cm^3}$
α	4	cm^{-1}
δ	0.04	–

The mass per area of 0.1 g/cm² is realistic. The factor $1.58\cdot10^9$ is defined to give 20 kHz as the maximum audible frequency. α is defined from the fact that 3.5 cm of BM length do have space for 10 octaves. The main friction stems from the hair cell and lymph film between OC and TM and is interactively adjusted by the value of δ.

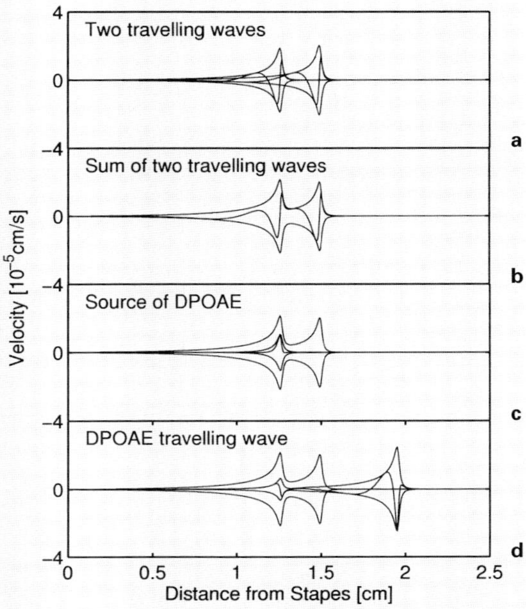

Fig. 2. a Velocity of BM oscillation for harmonic input of 1,000 and 1,600 Hz. The tonotopy principle is visible by the fact that the higher frequency wave cannot intrude so far toward the apex as the lower. **b** Sum of the two incoming traveling waves representing the stimulus for DPOAE generation. **c** The source term of the cubic DPOAE $2f_1 - f_2$ consists of $v_1^2 v_2^*$ and is located near the characteristic site of the incoming frequency f_2. The amplitude is enlarged by an arbitrary factor. **d** The traveling wave of frequency $2f_1 - f_2$ generated by the source term of **c**. It consists of one part traveling 'up', which can be heard, and one part traveling to the stapes, which eventually can be recorded in the ear canal.

the one which can be heard by trained, well-hearing people as the cubic difference tone of psychoacoustics, and (2) a wave traveling to the stapes, which eventually can be recorded in the outer ear canal. See figure 2 for some snapshots of the elements of this calculation. Again an animated view on computer screen is more impressive and particularly the role of the phases cannot be accounted for by written text or a snapshot picture.

On the basis of these fundamental calculations, we coupled a rather simple middle ear model together with a plugged ear canal model to the system. Then we studied their influence on the recordings of DPOAE as a function of frequency (fig. 3, 4). Two points might be stressed here, because they could be of clinical relevance: (1) near to the resonance frequency of the ear canal we possibly have to expect large differences in sound pressure level between eardrum and probe plug, and (2) the overall frequency dependence for the stiffness- or C-type nonlinearity, rolling off steeply with increasing frequency, favors the type of (possibly negative) friction- or R-type nonlinearity.

Discussion

We found that de Boer's linear model used as a basis for first order perturbation calculations: (1) does deliver cubic DPOAEs; (2) shows a unique source for the DP of frequency $2\omega_1 - \omega_2$ localized near the characteristic place of ω_2; (3) explains clearly that the further cubic distortion frequencies $2\omega_2 - \omega_1$, $3\omega_1$, $2\omega_1 + \omega_2$, $\omega_1 + 2\omega_2$, and $3\omega_2$ will have sources and will be generated within their 'forbidden region', and therefore cannot reach the stapes and the outer ear canal and consequently are missing in the registrations of DPOAE; (4) delivers a more realistic frequency dependency of L_{dp} if we use nonlinearity in friction instead of elasticity, and (5) allows for studies of the influence of middle ear, outer ear canal, and probe plug on the registrations.

On the other hand, there remain some problems: (1) The quoted calculations do not lead to a realistic level dependency of the DPOAEs, the function $L_{dp} = f(L_1,L_2)$. The experimental observation that to a fixed L_2 there is an optimum L_1 in the sense that still higher L_1 yields less L_{dp}, is not explained by first order perturbation calculation. It surely is a consequence of two-tone suppression, which cannot be cared for in the model before second order. (2) The well-known optimum of DP generation for an ω_2/ω_1 ratio of 1.2 is not explained by first order perturbation calculation, because it also must be a consequence of two-tone suppression. (3) The second DP source at the more apical characteristic site for $2\omega_1 - \omega_2$, which some experts require to explain the frequency depending fine structure of L_{dp}, would not appear before the fourth order perturbation. (The only contributing term consists of v_1^3 in the above sequence of DEs.) Nevertheless, it could deliver an outgoing wave large enough in amplitude to interfere with the first order outgoing wave. (4) There is no way in the simple model to give an account for the effect of additional suppressor tones, because two-tone suppression does not come in before second order perturbation.

Putting aside the problems 'ω_2/ω_1-ratio dependency', 'second source' and 'effect of suppressor tones' we discuss now the level dependence $L_{dp} = f(L_1,L_2)$. In a linear, inhomogeneous DE the size of the solution is proportional to the source term. In first order perturbation calculation the source term for the DPOAE of frequency $2\omega_1 - \omega_2$ is proportional to $v_{\omega 1}^2(x) \cdot v_{\omega 2}^*(x)$. Due to the square of $v_{\omega 1}^2(x)$ a

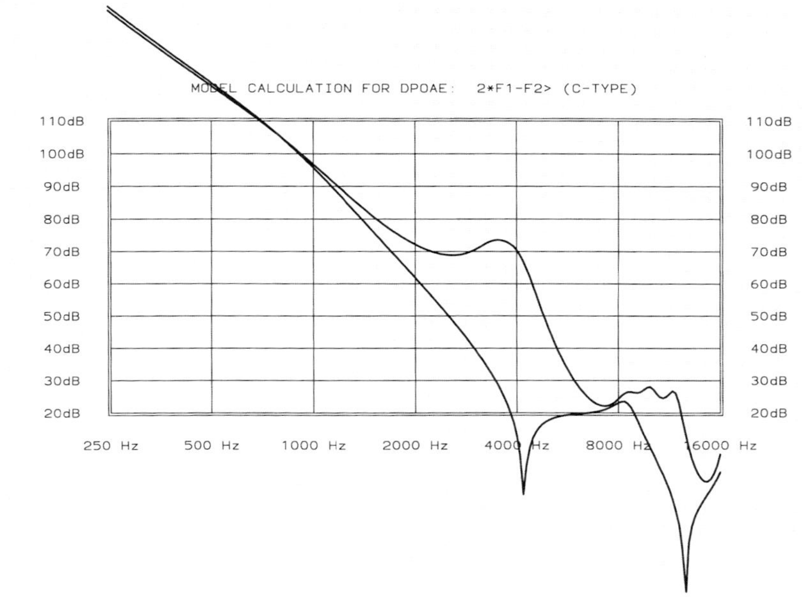

Fig. 3. The function $L_{dp}(\omega)$ calculated for a nonlinear elasticity in the simple model yields a drastic decrease of DPOAE levels over the commonly used frequency range. In comparison with experimental findings this does not seem realistic. The upper line shows the level at the eardrum while the lower line is the level at the earplug. The difference is a consequence of the ear canal resonance. Vertical scale is in arbitrary log values. [Modified from ref. 5.]

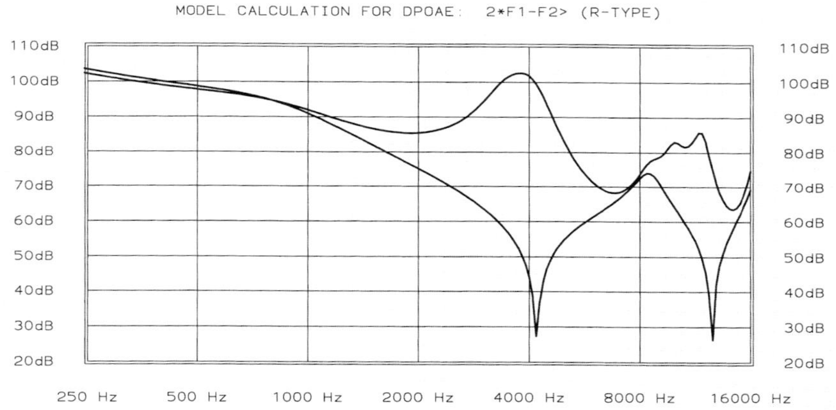

Fig. 4. The function $L_{dp}(\omega)$ calculated for a nonlinear friction in the simple model yields rather equal DPOAE levels over the commonly used frequency range. This is in good agreement with real measurements on human ears. The upper line shows the level at the eardrum while the lower line is the level at the earplug. The large difference is a consequence of the ear canal resonance. Vertical scale is in arbitrary log values. [Modified from ref. 5.]

decrease of L_1 by 5 dB must lower L_{dp} by 10 dB. Due to the fact that $v^*_{\omega 2}(x)$ is linear in the source term, a decrease of L_2 by 5 dB diminishes also L_{dp} by 5 dB. For the typical dynamic range of DPOAE registrations from (L_1, L_2) = (65 dB_{SPL}, 65 dB_{SPL}) down to (L_1, L_2) = (45 dB_{SPL}, 20 dB_{SPL}) this means a very large decrement of ΔL_{dp} = 85 dB in the model L_{dp}. (ΔL1 of 20 dB gives 40 dB, ΔL2 of 45 dB gives additional 45 dB.)

Experimental data, however, do show a decrease of *only 13 dB* over the same range: pointing to a strong nonlinear compression. Therefore, near the low level end some mechanism must deliver 72 dB increase in L_{dp} or at the high level end some other mechanism must cut the L_{dp} by 72 dB. This could be due to two reasons: (1) the problem might be not so weakly nonlinear as to be sufficiently described by first order perturbation calculation, and we had to make the effort to go to higher orders in ε, and (2) the shape and amplitude of the primary incoming waves do depend strongly on input level, and the incoming waves without any level dependence of shape are not adequate.

Actually the latter is already known from many experimental studies [8–10]. The incoming waves are of a sharply peaked form for low input levels, and of a more rounded form for high input levels. Besides, the maximum amplitudes show a strong compressive nonlinearity

Table 2. Model parameters of the improved model (step 2)

Parameter		
C_1	$1.58 \cdot 10^9 \cdot e^{-\alpha x}$	$\frac{dyn}{cm^3}$
M_1	0.1	$\frac{g}{cm^2}$
R_1	$0.03 \cdot \delta \sqrt{C_1 M_1}$	$\frac{dyn \cdot s}{cm^3}$
C_2	$1.58 \cdot 10^9 \cdot e^{-\alpha x}$	$\frac{dyn}{cm^3}$
M_2	0.05	$\frac{g}{cm^2}$
R_2	$0.03 \cdot \delta \sqrt{C_2 M_2}$	$\frac{dyn \cdot s}{cm^3}$
C_{12}	$0.001 \cdot C_1$	$\frac{dyn}{cm^3}$
R_{12}	$\delta \sqrt{C_1 M_1}$	$\frac{dyn \cdot s}{cm^3}$
α	4	cm^{-1}
δ	1	–

when drawn as a function of input level at stapes. The cochlea does compress the large dynamic range of acoustic pressure variations that enter the inner ear at the stapes, into the much smaller dynamic range that can be processed by sensory hair cells. According to experimental results [8, 9] the factor of this dynamic compression is about 3. So 25 dB dynamic range in amplitude of the incoming wave at their characteristic surging place is produced from 75 dB input range at the stapes.

Step 2

Modification of de Boer's model by implementation of a second degree of freedom in the organ of Corti.

Method

We can actually not expect that higher order corrections in cubic perturbation will compensate for the fault to have used unrealistic incoming waves in the lower orders before. Therefore we must find a new – possibly linear – operator Z_0 of a more complicated, maybe input level-dependent form, which delivers incoming waves with a realistic level dependency of form and amplitude. We can hope that, once the new Z_0 shapes realistic incoming waves, first order perturbation calculation alone will deliver a much better $L_{dp} = f(L_1, L_2)$ function. We follow a hint of J.B. Allen [pers. commun.] when we introduce a second degree of freedom for each cochlear partition of the model. As an expansion of the simple de Boer model we take into account movements of the tectorial membrane (TM) independent to some degree from the organ of Corti (OC). At a certain place x in the cochlea, the TM can make a radial movement and an up-down movement. We integrate the up-down movement into the up-down movement of the BM and the OC, but we do not restrict the radial movement. Radially the TM is coupled by friction and elasticity of the hair cells only to the movement of the OC. (By the way, in view of the visosity of the lymphatic film between TM and OC, it is of course not necessary that the hair tips are fixed at the TM.) The well-known shearing movement between TM and OC can then be *diminished*, when the TM is taken along *in phase* to the OC movement, but it can also be *enhanced*, when it is *in counter phase*. Phase relations of oscillations can be influenced by tuning the relative resonance properties of TM and OC.

So we need only to form an oscillator of the TM having the 'normal' characteristic frequency as a function of x and give the OC a slightly lower resonance frequency. If the latter can be changed, e.g. by slow motility tension of the outer hair cells, we will have a local filter which can be adjusted to have better or worse Q-value and higher or lower maximum amplitude. In the model we shall describe the mistuning between TM and OC by a local (or global) function $\eta(x)$. Clearly adjustment of the Q-value of the local partition must be able to modify the form of the traveling wave from a more round to a more peaked type. In Appendix 3 we derive the mathematical form for a Z_0 operator taking into account Allen's idea. For simplicity we do already here the conversion to frequency representation. The result for one frequency ω is:

$$z_0 = z_1 + \frac{z_2 \cdot z_{12}}{z_2 + z_{12}} = z_1 + z_2 \| z_{12}$$

Here the z are no longer operators but eigenvalues and in detail

$$z_1 = j\omega \cdot M_1 + R_1(x) - \frac{j}{\omega} \cdot C_1(x)$$

represents the OC and BM oscillator. It can be rewritten to:

$$z_1 = j\omega \cdot M_1 \cdot \left[1 - j \cdot 2\delta \cdot \frac{\omega_1(x)}{\omega} - \frac{\omega_1^2(x)}{\omega^2} \right]$$

$$= j\omega \cdot M_1 \cdot \left[1 - j \cdot 2\delta \cdot \frac{\omega_2(x) \cdot \eta(x)}{\omega} - \frac{(\omega_2(x) \cdot \eta(x))^2}{\omega^2} \right]$$

In the latter form the mistuning function $\eta(x)$ is explicitly contained. In a similar fashion the TM oscillator is given by:

$$z_2 = j\omega \cdot M_2 + R_2(x) - \frac{j}{\omega} \cdot C_2(x) = j\omega \cdot M_2 \cdot \left[1 - j \cdot 2 \cdot \delta_2 \cdot \frac{\omega_2(x)}{\omega} - \frac{\omega_2^2(x)}{\omega^2} \right]$$

and

$$z_{12} = R_{12}(x) - \frac{j}{\omega} \cdot C_{12}(x)$$

describes the coupling between TM and OC by friction and elasticity of the hair cells.

The new 'operator' z_0 is again linear. The constants herein are listed in table 2. The most important parameter $\eta(x)$, smaller than 1, is the ratio ω_1/ω_2 of the local resonance frequencies of OC and TM. Instead of adjusting it globally as a function of input level at stapes, we do the tuning of OC locally as a feedback function of the difference velocity between TM and OC. This seems to be physiologically

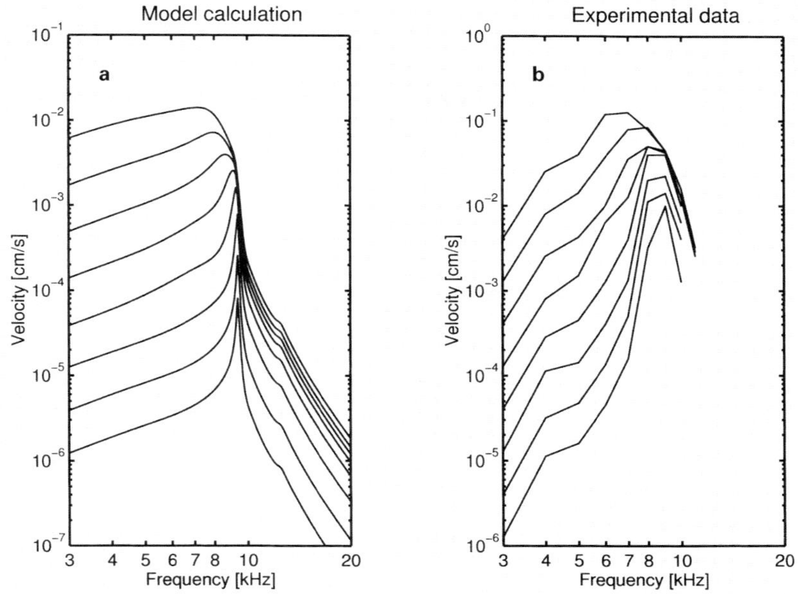

Fig. 5. a BM velocity amplitude at various constant sound pressure levels (from 80 to 10 dB SPL). The model velocity functions $|v_\omega(x)|$ for fixed frequency have been transformed to response functions $|v_x(\omega)|$ at fixed distance x = 3.5 mm from stapes in order to allow comparison to **b** experimental frequency response data at the same levels taken from Ruggero et al. [10]. The step 2 model can qualitatively model the typical sequence of response functions.

more plausible for a quick feedback. Because we do not want to make the mathematical problem strongly nonlinear, we perform the feedback by iteration:

(1) Set a standard start $\eta(x)$ function.
(2) Calculate p(x,t) and from it v(x,t).
(3) Calculate the difference velocity $v_{IHC}(x,t)$ from v(x,t).
(4) Calculate a new $\eta(x)$.
(5) Go to 2 twenty times.

Details of the feedback function can be found in Appendix 4. This function locally adjusts the elasticity of the BM in dependence on the membrane's motion itself.

Results

Using the model parameter set of table 2 we again produced 'incoming waves' $v_\omega(x)$ for fixed frequencies ω as function of x. They can be transformed to frequency response functions $v_x(\omega)$ for fixed x as functions of frequency. So we can compare them to experimental data of Ruggero et al. [10] in figure 5. The wave shaping strong nonlinearity, which consists in the recursive adaptation of the mistuning function $\eta(x)$, does not quite exactly reproduce the experimental data, but the main features of compressive nonlinearity and drift of the maximum response frequency are correct. Besides, for low input levels the functions contain a sharp peak near the characteristic frequency, which first diminishes and later disappears as input level goes up. We remember: the source term for the DPOAE of frequency $2\omega_1 - \omega_2$ is proportional to $v^2_{\omega_1}(x) \cdot v^*_{\omega_2}(x)$. The shape of $v^2_{\omega_1}(x)$ at its basal slope is not influenced strongly by the feedback, while its size here grows according to twice L_1. On the other hand, the shape and size of $v_{\omega_2}(x)$ change considerably by the feedback. Therefore, we can expect that only the compressive dynamic of $v_{\omega_2}(x)$ is quantitatively 'mirrored out' to the ear canal via DP generation.

Now in the possession of well-shaped incoming waves we could try to reprdocue the $L_{dp} = f(L_1,L_2)$ function. Figure 6 gives an equal L_{dp} contour plot fitted to experimental data of nine normal ears measured for 18 frequencies at 16 level pairs (L_1,L_2). It exhibits a sort of shoulder with the optimum line for clinical measurements. Without any additional optimization, our DPOAE model delivers a quite similar contour plot (fig. 7). We have to admit, however, that the total compression is not yet reproduced.

We regard a cross-sectional view of the OC. Plausibly a contraction of the outer hair cells would turn the Ductus endolymphaticus slightly radially and downwards, at the same time rising the local tension of the BM and its local resonance frequency. That exactly is what our mistuning function $\eta(x)$ could do. We get some support for this speculative idea by a comparison of our calculation to an experimental study of LePage [11]. Figure 8 faces a diagram of LePage with a corresponding model calculation. While the frequency response function of the model resembles the experimental one, the $\eta(x)$ is similar to the static displacement as measured by LePage.

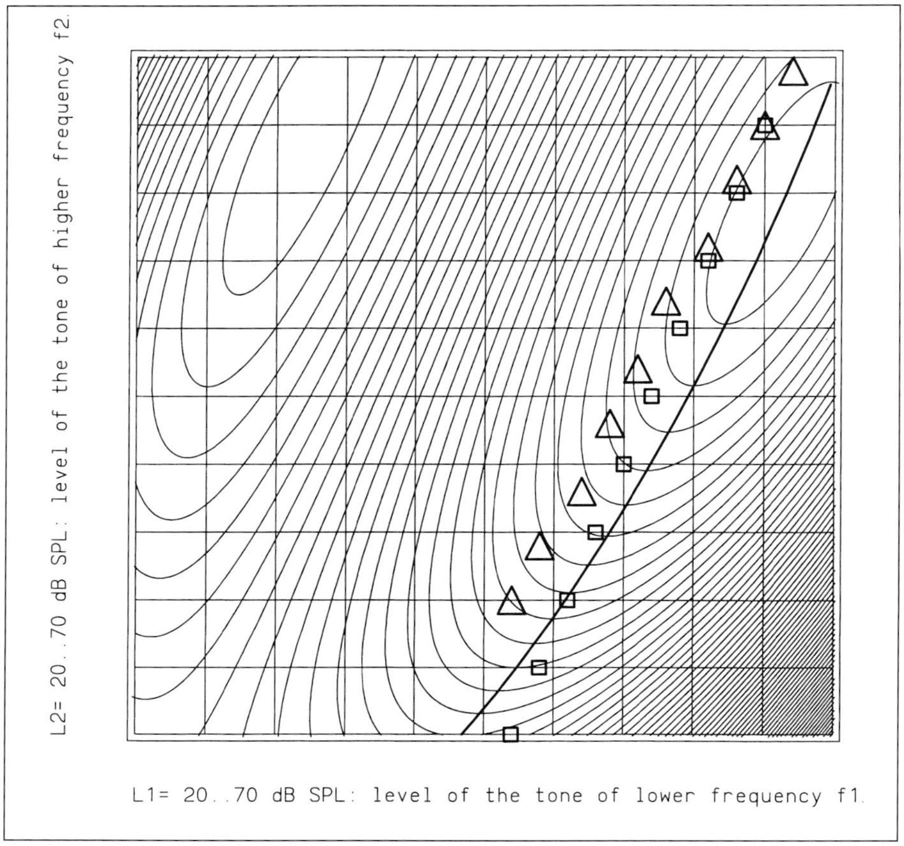

Fig. 6. Bi-cubic surface fit for Ldp = f(L1,L2). Experimental data were taken from 9 ears, at 18 frequencies from 8 kHz down to 1 kHz, at 16 properly distributed level pairs (L1, L2). The distance of the grid lines is 5 dB. The level contours are in 1-dB steps. The slightly bent fat line running down the 'shoulder' would give the ideal (L1, L2) pairs. Squares give the 10 level pairs optimized according to Männlein-Mangold [5], triangles give the 'level scissors' after Janssen et al. [7]. Due to a very strong compressive nonlinearity along the ideal line, one counts only 13 dB dynamic for L_{dp}. [Modified from ref. 5.]

Discussion

In step 1, with relatively small effort we found that the use of de Boer's linear 1-D model as a basis for first order perturbation calculations: (1) Does actually deliver cubic DPOAEs. (2) Shows an unequivocal source for the DP of frequency $2\omega_1 - \omega_2$ localized near the characteristic place of ω_2. (3) Explains clearly that the further cubic distortion frequencies $2\omega_2 - \omega_1$, $3\omega_1$, $2\omega_1 + \omega_2$, $\omega_1 + 2\omega_2$, and $3\omega_2$ will have sources, but will be generated within their 'forbidden region'. This means no generation of additional *traveling* waves. Therefore these frequencies cannot reach the stapes and the outer ear canal, and consequently are missing in the registrations. (4) Delivers a more realistic frequency dependency of L_{dp} if we use nonlinearity in friction instead of elasticity. (5) Allows for studies of the influence of middle ear, outer ear canal, and probe plug on the registrations.

In step 2 we have developed a more complicated version of our mathematical model of DPOAE generation by inclusion of a second degree of freedom in the cochlear partition. The TM can radially move freely and is coupled to the motion of the BM mainly by the strong friction of the hair cells. By fine tuning the local resonance frequency of the BM in relation to the local resonance frequency of the TM oscillator we have a local filter of adjustable Q-value. So the primary incoming waves can be shaped in a realistic way, and serve as a well-adapted raw material to construct the source term for DPOAE generation. The challenge of course was to let the incoming waves perform the tuning of the filter and the reshaping by feedback automatically: The results will be repropted later.

The progress over step 1 now is: (1) The experimental level function $L_{dp} = f(L_1,L_2)$ can be reproduced qualitatively, though not quantitatively. (2) Still the exact quantitative behavior, in particular the high compression factor, needs additional fine adjustment of the feedback algorithm. (3) The two-tone suppression does work in principle, but quantitatively it is not yet strong enough. (4) For the reproduction of the $L_{dp} = f(\omega_2/\omega_1)$ function we will have to change the strongly nonlinear feedback mechanism.

Conclusion

Looking back we can be content that starting with a rather simple model we were able to illuminate some of the secrets of DPOAE generation. The effort grew with the wish to be more quantitative. There exist, however, some interesting challenges in the adaptation and adjustment of the model. Beside fundamental understanding of DPOAE generation we hope to deliver the more clinical aspects of pathologic function as well.

For the moment the most urging need seems to be a more realistic mechanism of two-tone suppression possibly having its solution in an optimized $\eta(x)$ function. Figure 9 gives the present state: While f2 is stepped towards f1 the two peaks in BM velocity envelope do not break down as much as a real suppression would request. Instead they still sum up too much. It might be necessary, beside the mistuning function, also to implement a dynamically adjustable, possibly negative, friction within the improved Z_0, particularly in the z_{12} part. It can be implemented in the 1-D model and there is no reason why $L_{dp} = f(L_1, L_2)$ should not be further improved, and no reason why $L_{dp} = f(\omega_2/\omega_1)$ should not show the well-known optimum for $\omega_2/\omega_1 = 1.2$. Additional suppressor tones will then be no problem. All this will be step 3. Once having the proper feedback-shaped incoming waves we will

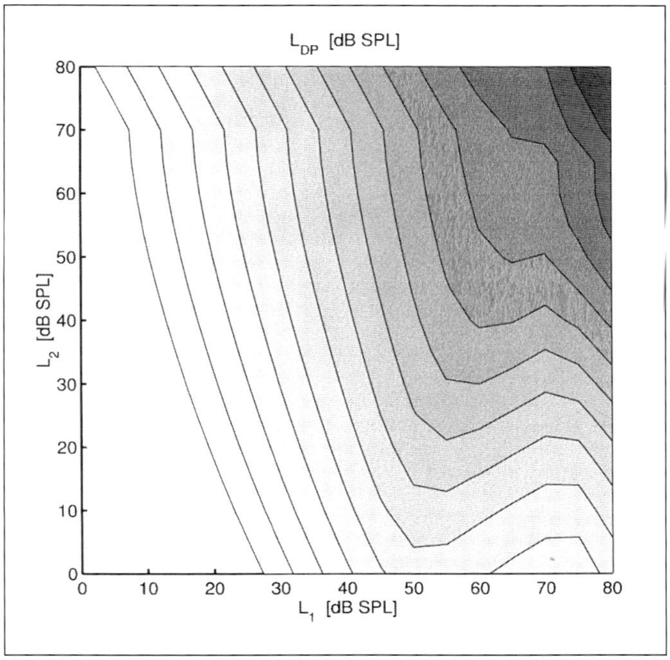

Fig. 7. Surface contour plot calculated by the step 2 model. Without further adjustment of $\eta(x)$ the model yields a quite realistic shoulder form in $L_{dp} = f(L_1, L_2)$. Still however, the compression is not high enough. The calculated dynamic in Ldp corresponding to figure 6 still is as large as 45 dB. Remember however that the step 1 model delivers 85 dB for the same input range. [Modified from ref. 6.]

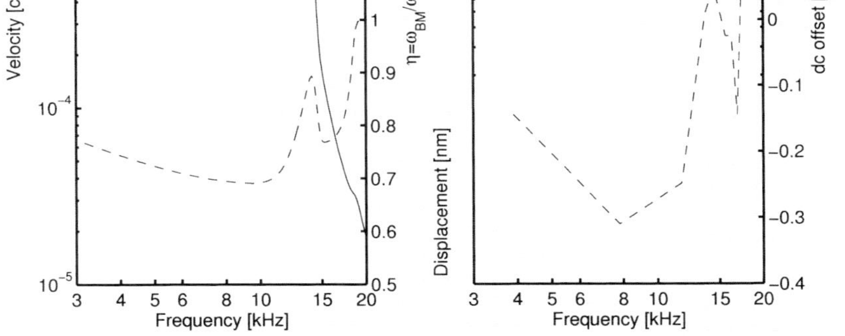

Fig. 8. a Calculated basilar membrane velocity envelope (solid line), transformed to a site with the characteristic frequency = 15.6 kHz and the corresponding function $\eta(x)$ (dashed line) for input level L = 70 dB SPL. **b** Experimental data from LePage [11] for the same input level. The solid line is the displacement when the cochlea is stimulated with a harmonic tone. The 'dc offset' (dashed line) has been measured at the place of CF = 15.6 kHz and describes a deformation of the organ of Corti.

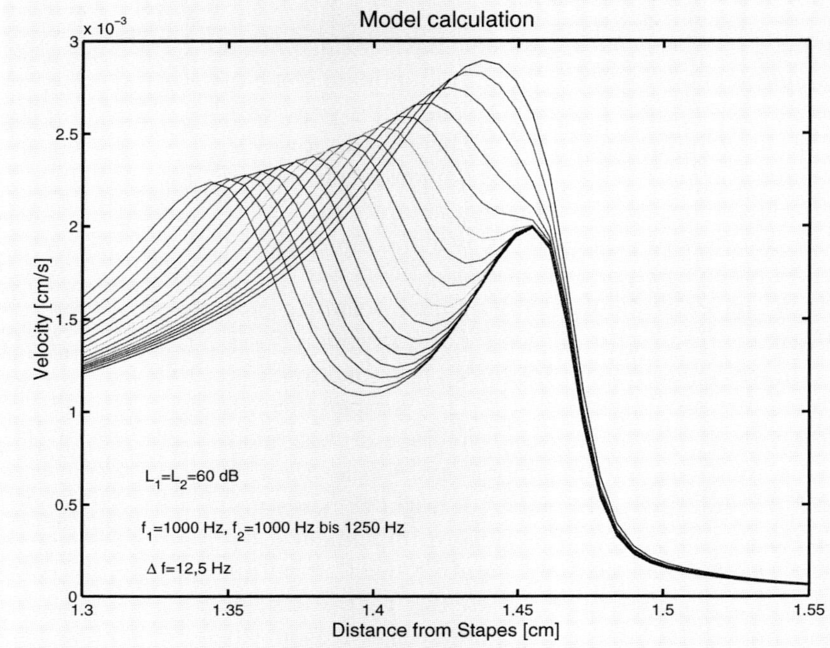

Fig. 9. Still not satisfying state of the two-tone suppression of the model: The higher pitched tone is stepped down from 1,250 to 1,000 Hz, the frequency of the lower pitched tone. The peak amplitude of the higher tone should be stepwise depressed in a much higher degree. Steps 3 and 4 will modify the model to adopt this. The total compression in $L_{dp} = f(L_1,L_2)$, the optimum in $L_{dp} = f(\omega_2/\omega_1)$, and, of course, the effect of further suppressor tones will not be reporduced by the model before two-tone suppression is implemented in a more realistic way.

go to higher orders of perturbation calculation in step 4. Modeling of the suppression of the interfering second source in particular will be interesting.

Acknowledgments

The authors both are working in the clinical field and have to thank for the daily challenges of clinical relevance. They apologize for shortly being on a detour and promise that the outcomes will deliver a proper understanding of the mechanisms of normal and pathological DPOAE generation not before long.

The authors feel gratefully indebted to many colleagues giving ongoing contributions to this work. Hellmut von Specht has given decisive impacts in many interesting discussions with one of us (M.G.) to this and the foregoing studies. Thomas Hocke has constructed and built the sophisticated measuring equipment and Katrin Mentzel has performed most of the measurements in Magdeburg. Many of the ideas herein stem from discussions with Margarete Männlein-Mangold, when she prepared her thesis with M.B. in Erlangen. She was also kindly supported by Ute Pröschel, Sebastian Hoth and Thomas Janssen. Horst Letz has given valuable help regarding mathematical methods. J.B. Allen, on a short visit to Munich, gave the definitive hint regarding the TM-BM coupling. Lothar U. Kohllöffel has contributed his detailed knowledge of the inner ear of nearly any species in the world and helped us to define some of the model parameters in a realistic way. Hanns Ruder some decades ago taught one of us (M.B.) to make mathematical models in an essential way, to interpret them and to mind their limits.

Appendices

Appendix 1: Some Remarks on How to Solve the DEs

We can reduce the partial DEs to simple ones by expanding all functions into frequency eigenfunction:

$$p(x,t) = \sum_{\omega} P_{\omega}(x)\cdot|\omega\rangle$$

$$u(x,t) = \sum_{\omega} u_{\omega}(x)\cdot|\omega\rangle$$

$$v(x,t) = \sum_{\omega} v_{\omega}(x)\cdot|\omega\rangle$$

Here $|\omega\rangle = e^{j\omega t}$ and has the comfortable properties

$$\frac{d}{dt}|\omega\rangle = j\omega\cdot|\omega\rangle \text{ and } \int dt|\omega\rangle = -\frac{j}{\omega}\cdot|\omega\rangle$$

which convert the t-operators to simple numbers. We insert these Fourier series expansions into the DE and from

$$Z_0 v(x,t) = M\cdot\frac{d}{dt}v(x,t) + R(x)\cdot v(x,t) + C(x)\cdot\int v(x,t)dt =$$

$$\sum_{\omega} (j\omega\cdot M + R(x) - \frac{j}{\omega}C(x))\cdot v_{\omega}(x)\cdot|\omega\rangle$$

abbreviating

$$j\omega\cdot M + R(x) - \frac{j}{\omega}C(x) = z_0$$

we get

$$\sum_{\omega}[z_0\cdot v_\omega(x) + 2p_\omega(x)]\cdot|\omega\rangle = 0.$$

We apply $\langle\omega'|$ and because of $\langle\omega'|\omega\rangle = \delta^{\omega}_{\omega'}$, get rid of the summation:

$$z_0\cdot v_\omega(x) + 2p_\omega(x) = 0 \qquad (**)$$

The inertia of the periplymph fluid of density ρ gives the equation:

$$\frac{d}{dt}u(x,t) = -\frac{1}{\rho}\cdot\frac{\partial}{\partial x}p(x,t)$$

The continuity or incompressibility of perilymph fluid in a scala of effective height H gives another equation:

$$\frac{\partial}{\partial x}u(x,t) = -\frac{1}{H}\cdot v(x,t)$$

By combination of these two DEs we can eliminate u(x,t) and find:

$$-\frac{1}{\rho}\cdot\frac{\partial^2}{\partial x^2}p(x,t) = \frac{1}{H}\cdot\frac{d}{dt}\cdot v(x,t),$$

which by Fourier transform delivers:

$$v_\omega(x) = \frac{j}{\omega}\cdot\frac{H}{\rho}\cdot\frac{\partial^2}{\partial x^2}p_\omega(x).$$

We combine this with our DE (**) from above and find:

$$\frac{\partial^2}{\partial x^2}p_\omega(x) + \frac{2\rho}{M\cdot H}\cdot\frac{1}{1 - j\cdot\frac{R(x)}{\omega\cdot M} - \frac{1}{\omega^2}\cdot\frac{C(x)}{M}}\cdot p_\omega(x) = 0.$$

We introduce some abbreviations by the definitions:

$$\frac{C(x)}{M} = \frac{C_0\cdot e^{-2\alpha\cdot x}}{M} = \omega_0^2\cdot e^{-2\alpha\cdot x} \text{ and}$$

$$\frac{R(x)}{M} = \frac{2\cdot\delta\cdot\sqrt{C(x)\cdot M}}{M} = 2\cdot\delta\cdot\omega_0\cdot e^{-\alpha\cdot x}.$$

Our main DE now is:

$$\frac{\partial^2}{\partial x^2}p_\omega(x) + \frac{2p}{MH}\cdot\frac{1}{1-\frac{\omega_0^2}{\omega^2}\cdot e^{-2\alpha\cdot x} - j\cdot 2\delta\cdot\frac{\omega_0}{\omega}\cdot e^{-\alpha\cdot x}}\cdot p_\omega(x) = 0$$

Having solved this DE for $p_\omega(x)$ we can easily calculate $v_\omega(x)$ and $u_\omega(x)$.

The boundary conditions necessary to solve the linear second order DE are:

$p_\omega(x = 35\text{ mm}) = 0$;

$p_\omega(x = 0)$ = adapted to input level.

The algorithm to solve the DE consists in use of a discrete x-scale of 1,200 steps and a 5-point formula for $\partial^2/\partial x^2$. We then finally have to solve an inhomogeneous (1,200 × 1,200) matrix equation with a matrix having only 5 diagonals.

The left-hand side of all DEs of the perturbation series is the same, except for the boundary conditions: The input comes only in order zero. For the higher orders, where we produce the distortion products and their higher order corrections, the boundary condition at stapes consists in the correct impedance of the plugged outer ear canal as seen through the middle ear by the inner ear: in effect a certain frequency-dependent gvalue for the ratio of

$$p_\omega(x = 0)/\frac{\partial}{\partial x}p_\omega(x = 0).$$

Appendix 2: Calculation of the Source Terms

The right-hand side of the DE series needs some more treatment: Typically the incoming waves $v_0(x,t)$ do contain two frequency components $|\omega_1\rangle$ and $|\omega_2\rangle$. To keep them as real functions we have to include also their two complex conjugates $|-\omega_1\rangle$ and $|-\omega_2\rangle$. Therefore, the right-hand side in first order perturbation theory for the frictional or R-type perturbation is written as:

$$-Z_1v_0(x,t) =$$
$$-R\cdot(v_{\omega_1}(x)\cdot|\omega_1\rangle + v_{\omega_2}(x)\cdot|\omega_2\rangle + v^*_{\omega_1}(x)\cdot|-\omega_1\rangle + v^*_{\omega_2}(x)\cdot|\omega_2\rangle)^3.$$

If the $(...)^3$ is expanded, it delivers eight different frequency components:

$$3\cdot v^2_{\omega_1}(x)\cdot v^*_{\omega_2}(x)\cdot|2\omega_1 - \omega_2\rangle,$$
$$[3\cdot v_{\omega_1}(x)\cdot v^*_{\omega_1}(x) + 6\cdot v_{\omega_2}(x)\cdot v^*_{\omega_2}(x)]\cdot v_{\omega_1}(x)\cdot|\omega_1\rangle,$$
$$[6\cdot v_{\omega_1}(x)\cdot v^*_{\omega_1}(x) + 3\cdot v_{\omega_2}(x)\cdot v^*_{\omega_2}(x)]\cdot v_{\omega_2}(x)\cdot|\omega_2\rangle,$$
$$3\cdot v^*_{\omega_1}(x)\cdot v^2_{\omega_2}(x)\cdot|2\omega_2 - \omega_1\rangle,$$
$$v^3_{\omega_1}(x)\cdot|3\omega_1\rangle,$$
$$3\cdot v^2_{\omega_1}(x)\cdot v_{\omega_2}(x)\cdot|2\omega_1+\omega_2\rangle,$$
$$3\cdot v_{\omega_1}(x)\cdot v^2_{\omega_2}(x)\cdot|2_{\omega_2}+\omega_1\rangle,$$
$$v^3_{\omega_2}(x)\cdot|3_{\omega_2}\rangle$$

and their conjugate complex forms.

Because we solve the DEs in the frequency domain some $\langle\omega'|$ operation has to be performed on the left- and on the right-hand sides of the DEs. Here 'hits', sources different from zero, will be found only for the eight mentioned frequencies and their negatives. For example the source term for the generation of the most important DP frequency of $|2\omega_1 - \omega_2\rangle$ comes out as $-R\cdot 3\cdot v^2_{\omega_1}(x)\cdot v^*_{\omega_2}(x)$ in the frictional nonlinearity. For the nonlinear elasticity or 'c-type' the source term has an additional frequency denominator stemming from the time integration:

$$-\frac{C(x)}{(2\omega_1 - \omega_2)^3}\cdot 3\cdot v^2_{\omega_1}(x)\cdot v^*_{\omega_2}(x).$$

It is this denominator, by the way, which cuts down the L_{dp} drastically with increasing frequency (see fig. 3). It must be acknowledged here that the source terms in higher order do contain more and more frequency components and in fourth order practically cannot be evaluated by hand.

Appendix 3: The Improved Z_0

For the solution we go to the frequency representation and do all calculations for one frequency ω after the other. We regard the OC as one oscillator described by the 'vertical' velocity $v_\omega(x)$ and driven by the local difference pressure between scala vestibuli and scala tympani. The TM in vertical direction simply is taken away also by $v_\omega(x)$, thus increasing the mass M_1 and possibly R_1 and C_1. The radial oscillatory motion of the TM is designated by the function $w_\omega(x)$. Disregarding a constant factor (which readily can be drawn into M_2, R_2 and C_2) $w_\omega(x) - v_\omega(x)$ is the shearing velocity of OC against TM, which is the input for the hair cells. The coupling between TM and OC oscillators is performed by strong friction and weak elasticity of the hair cells and the 5-µm-thick endolymph film. The motion of the two oscillators is described by:

$$(j\omega \cdot M_1 + R_1 - \frac{j}{\omega} C_1) v_\omega = -2p_\omega + (-\frac{j}{\omega} C_{12} + R_{12})(w_\omega - v_\omega) \qquad (1')$$

which in short is:

$$z_1 \cdot v_\omega = -2p_\omega + z_{12} \cdot (w_\omega - v_\omega) \qquad (1)$$

and by:

$$(j\omega \cdot M_2 + R_2 - \frac{j}{\omega} C_2) w_\omega = (-\frac{j}{\omega} C_{12} + R_{12})(v_\omega - w_\omega) \qquad (2')$$

which again in short is:

$$z_2 \cdot w_\omega = z_{12} \cdot (v_\omega - w_\omega) \qquad (2)$$

From (2) we can express ω_ω by v_ω:

$$w_\omega = \frac{z_{12}}{z_2 + z_{12}} \cdot v_\omega$$

and can replace w_ω in (1):

$$(z_1 + \frac{z_2 \cdot z_{12}}{z_2 + z_{12}}) \cdot v_\omega = -2p_\omega.$$

If we remember that z, v and p are dependent on x, we have the brackets on the left-hand side as our new, improved Z_0. It is transformed already to ω representation and so consisting only of its eigenvalues.

Appendix 4: How Does η(x) Depend on the Movement of TM and OC?

The hair cell input signal in our improved model is the difference of w and v. It easily is calculated to be:

$$v_{IHC} = \sum_\omega v_\omega - w_\omega = \sum_\omega \left(1 - \frac{z_{12}}{z_2 + z_{12}}\right) \cdot v_\omega = \sum_\omega \left(\frac{z_2}{z_2 + z_{12}}\right) \cdot v_\omega$$

The sum has to be extended over all incoming frequencies. (We remember that the z, w and the v do depend on x.) The relative mistuning η(x) between the local TM and OC resonance is calculated from a former guess v_{IHC} by the relation:

$$\eta(x) = \begin{cases} \eta_{max} \text{ for } v_{IHC}(x) < v_{min} & \text{case a} \\ \eta_{min} \text{ for } v_{IHC}(x) > v_{max} & \text{case b} \\ \eta_{min} + \dfrac{\log(|v_{IHC}(x)|/v_{max})}{\log(v_{min}/v_{max})} \cdot (\eta_{max} - \eta_{min}) & \text{else.} \end{cases}$$

It is essential that η(x) is a nonlinear function of v_{IHC}, because of the conditions a and b. The parameters for this central feedback function need an interactive fine adjustment, and possibly a different form of this function will be more appropriate. We remember for example the fact that the innervation of the OHCs are coupled for about 1 mm in x direction and therefore smooth this η(x) over a range of 1 mm before we apply it for the next calculation of the different v_ω and the new v_{IHC}, respectively. We could not only produce more realistic incoming waves, as for their level dependence, but we also can expect that basically two-tone suppression is automatically contained in this way.

References

1 de Boer E: Auditory physics: Physical principles in hearing theory. I. Phys Rep 1980;62:87–174.
2 Neely ST, Kim DO: A model for active elements in cochlear biomechanics. J Acoust Soc Am 1986;79:1472–1480.
3 Allen JB: A cochlear micromechanic model of transduction; in van den Brink G, Bilsen FA (eds): Psychophysical, Physiological and Behavioural Studies in Hearing. Delft, Delft University Press, 1980, pp 85–95.
4 Ganz M, Berg M: Modellierung otoakustischer Verzerrungsprodukte unter Verwendung der Methode der Störungsrechnung. Z Audiol 1998 (suppl I):29–30.
5 Männlein-Mangold M: Otoakustisch emittierte Distorsionsprodukte; Diss, Erlangen-Nürnberg 1998.
6 Ganz M: Theoretische und experimentelle Untersuchungen zur Innenohrmechanik unter Anwendung otoakustischer Verzerrungsprodukte; Diss, Magdeburg 1999.
7 Janssen T, Kummer P, Arnold W: Growth behavior of the 2f1–f2 distortion product otoacoustic emission in tinnitus. J Acoust Soc Am 1998;103:3418–3430.
8 Rhode WS: Observations of the vibrations of the basilar membrane in squirrel monkeys using the Mössbauer technique. J Acoust Soc Am 1971;49:1218–1231.
9 Johnstone BM, Patuzzi R, Yates GK: Basilar membrane measurements and the travelling wave. Hear Res 1986;22:147–153.
10 Ruggero MA, Rich NC, Recio A, Shyamla Narayan S, Robles L: Basilar-membrane responses to tones at the base of the chinchilla cochlea. J Acoust Soc Am 1997;101:2151–2163.
11 LePage EL: Frequency-dependent self-induced bias of the basilar membrane and its potential for controlling sensitivity and tuning in the mammalian cochlea. J Acoust Soc Am 1987;82:139–154.

ORL

ORL 1999;61:287–293

Nonlinear Electroelastic Model for the Composite Outer Hair Cell Wall

Alexander A. Spector

Department of Biomedical Engineering and Center for Computational Medicine and Biology, Johns Hopkins University, Baltimore, Md., USA

Key Words

Outer hair cell, model · Nonlinear shell · Active force

Abstract

A nonlinear electroelastic model for the composite wall of the cochlear outer hair cell is proposed. The cell wall is modeled as a two-layer shell with elastic connections between the layers: an active layer corresponds to the plasma membrane and a passive layer corresponds to a combination of the cytoskeleton and the subsurface cisternae. As a basis of the constitutive relations, a thermodynamic potential for such a composite wall is developed. Expressions for the components of the active force are obtained in terms of the active strains and the elastic properties of the passive and active layers. An application to the electrical stimulation of the cell under the conditions of the microchamber experiment is given. As a result, active strains, active forces, and mechanical energy stored in each of the two layers are presented as functions of the wall (membrane) potential.

Introduction

Outer hair cells play the major role in the active processes in the mammalian ear, providing it with amplification and fine frequency selectivity. As an element of hearing, outer hair cells are involved in a multistep process occurring at the organ, cellular, and subcellular levels. Two main parts of this process are mechanoelectrical transduction of the stereocilia bending into the receptor current and electromechanical transduction of the cell's wall potential changes into the length changes and the active force production. The two steps are accompanied by numerous events that involve both the components of the outer hair cells and the whole cochlea. Bending of the stereocilia is caused by relative motion of the basilar membrane, reticular lamina, and tectorial membrane. The transduction current is determined by the inclination of the stereocilia as well as the electrical gradient within the cochlea. The electromechanical transduction includes excitation of the molecular motors and transmission of the active forces and strains through the composite cell wall. This transduction involves the molecular components of the cell wall, such as actin filaments and spectrin crosslinks in the cytoskeleton and the protein particles and lipid bilayer in the plasma membrane.

The active processes in the cochlea are physiologically vulnerable, and the outer hair cells are especially susceptible to damage. The cell's performance can be severely affected by acoustic trauma, ototoxic drugs, and aging. Various forms of damage of the stereocilia have been found to accompany the action of acoustic trauma [1]. It has been recently shown that acoustic trauma results in a reduction of outer hair cell stiffness [2]. Salicylate is known to cause reversible hearing loss and tinnitus. Salic-

KARGER

Fax + 41 61 306 12 34
E-Mail karger@karger.ch
www.karger.com

© 1999 S. Karger AG, Basel
0301–1569/99/0615–0287$17.50/0

Accessible online at:
http://BioMedNet.com/karger

Alexander A. Spector, PhD
Department of Biomedical Engineering
Johns Hopkins University
Baltimore, MD 21205 (USA)
Tel. +1 410 502 6955, Fax +1 410 955 0549, E-Mail aspector@bme.jhu.edu

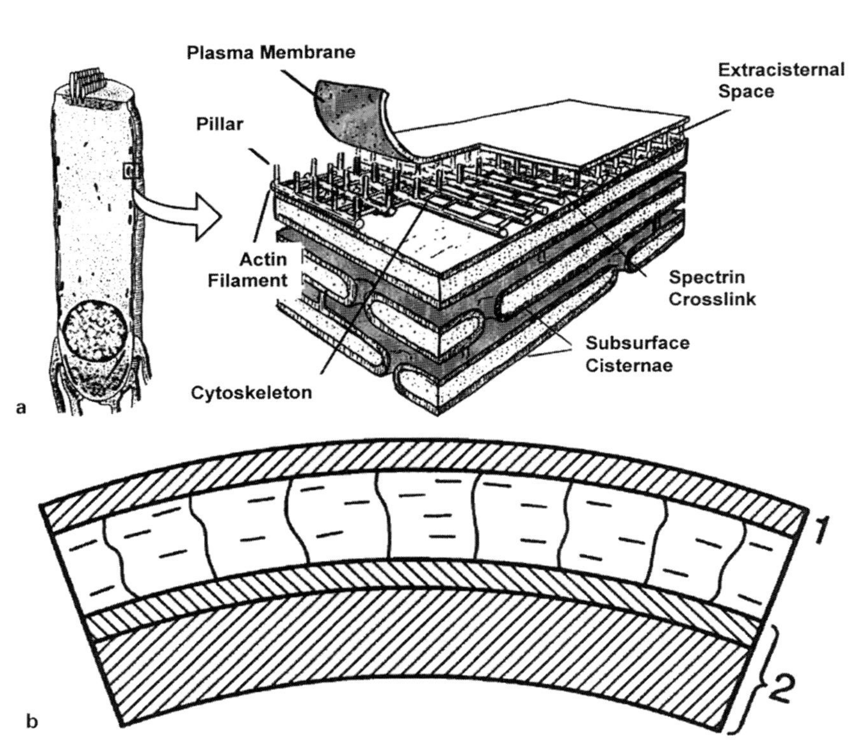

Fig. 1. General view of outer hair cell and the microstructure of the cell wall with the major components of the cell wall (**a**) and model of the composite cell wall (**b**).

ylate has a strong effect on the outer hair cell's electromotile and mechanical properties. Outer hair cells treated with salicylate lose their turgidity, a necessary element of the cell's normal behavior [3]. A reduction of the axial stiffness of outer hair cell treated with salicylate has been observed [4]. The micropipet aspiration experiment showed a similar reduction in the cell's radial stiffness [5]. Salicylate dramatically inhibits outer hair cell electromotility. Several independent groups [4, 6, 7] have reported a severalfold decrease in the electromotile response of salicylate-treated outer hair cells. It has also been shown [8] that this decrease is accompanied by a substantial reduction of the transferred charge and nonlinear capacitance of the cell. Quinine used therapeutically (e.g., for the treatment of malaria) has side effects related to a loss of hearing sensitivity. The effect of quinine on isolated outer hair cells has been studied and demonstrated to cause dramatic shape changes and cell death [9]. Aging-related sensorineural hearing impairment is accompanied by loss of outer hair cells located at the basal part of the cochlea. Aging-related pathological changes in the outer hair cell's properties and behavior have not been understood with certainty. One of the known pathological features of elderly people is atrophy of stria vascularis, which is thought to be the cause of slow progressive senorineural hearing loss [10]. A relation between degeneration of stria vascularis and decline of the endocochlear potential has been discovered [11]. The endocochlear potential determines the potential gradient inside the cochlea that drives outer hair cell electromotility. This finding [11] could help to establish an important connection between aging and decline of the electromotile properties of outer hair cells.

In the present paper, we propose a model that reflects major structural components of the composite outer hair cell wall as well as typical features of cell electromotility. We represent the wall as two layers with deformable connections between them. The outer layer (plasma membrane) is considered as an isotropic nonlinear electroelastic shell; the inner layer (a combination of the cytoskeleton and the subsurface cisternae) is considered as an orthotropic linear elastic shell, the connections (radial pillars) are represented by distributed elastic springs (fig. 1). Anisotropy (orthotropy) of the passive layer comes from the properties of the cytoskeleton made of two protein networks with different elastic and geometric characteristics. The present model is a development of our previous models of a single-layer electroelastic shell [12] and a composite three-layer elastic shell [13]. Our present model corresponds to the hypothesis of an active plasma membrane [14] with the transmission of the active strains and forces generated within it to the passive cytoskeleton and subsurface cisternae. We give an expression of the thermodynamic potential for such a composite and derive constitutive relations for each layer. We introduce the active strains to characterize the plasma membrane response to potential variation under the conditions of unchanged membrane stresses (resultant forces). We apply our model to the case of the outer hair cell's electrical stimulation under the conditions of the microchamber experiment and find expressions for the generated active forces in terms of the elastic properties of the components of the composite wall and the active strains. By using our previous estimates of the elastic moduli of the cell wall [15] and a Boltzmann-type approximation of the active force [12, 16], we give graphs for two components of the active force in terms of the wall (plasma membrane) potential. We also present graphs for elastic energy accumulated within the passive and active layers as a result of the electrical stimulation of the active layer. These graphs are given in terms of the wall (plasma membrane) potential for physiological ranges of elastic moduli of the passive layer.

Mathematical Model

To derive constitutive relations for the strains and resultant forces (bending moments) within both (passive and active) layers as well as the electric displacement within the active layer, we start with a general thermodynamic potential for the composite wall:

$$W = U_1 + U_2 + k_n(w^1 - w^2)^2 + k_x(u_x^1 - u_x^2)^2 + k_\theta(u_\theta^1 - u_\theta^2)^2 + f_x(\Delta\psi)\varepsilon_x^1 + f_\theta(\Delta\psi)\varepsilon_\theta^1 + G(\Delta\psi)$$

where U_1 and U_2 define, respectively, internal mechanical energy of the active and the passive layer; u_x^1, u_θ^1, and w^1 are the components of the displacement of the active layer; u_x^2, u_θ^2, and w^2 are the components of the displacement of the passive layer; k_n, k_x, k_θ are the stiffness coefficients of the pillars; ε_x^1 and ε_θ^1 are the components of the active layer strains; $f_x(\Delta\psi)$ and $f_\theta(\Delta\psi)$ are nonlinear functions of the wall (membrane) potential characterizing the membrane piezoelectric properties, and $G(\Delta\psi)$ is a function of the order higher than quadratic characterizing the membrane electrical properties. This function describes the permittivity of the membrane, and it can be determined by using experimental data of the membrane capacitance [17, 18]. The first five terms in the expression for W determine mechanical energy of the composite wall, including the plasma membrane, cytoskeleton, radial pillars, and subsurface cisternae. The next two terms determine nonlinear electromechanical coupling within the plasma membrane. The last term determines purely electrical energy of the plasma membrane.

The internal mechanical energy of the active layer modeled here as an isotropic shell has the following form [19]:

$$U_1 = 0.5[C_{11}^1(\varepsilon_x^1)^2 + 2C_{12}^1\varepsilon_x^1\varepsilon_\theta^1 + C_{11}^1(\varepsilon_\theta^1)^2] + 2G^1(\varepsilon_{x\theta}^1)^2 + 0.5[D_{11}^1(\kappa_x^1)^2 + 2D_{12}^1\kappa_x^1\kappa_\theta^1 + D_{11}^1(\kappa_\theta^1)^2] + 2D_\tau^1(\tau^1)^2$$

where C_{11}^1, C_{22}^1, and G^1 are isotropic in-plane moduli; D_{11}^1, D_{12}^1, and D_τ^1 are isotropic bending and twisting moduli; $\varepsilon_{x\theta}^1$ is the shear component of the strain, and κ_x^1, κ_θ^1, and τ^1 are the components of the curvature and twist changes of the plasma membrane.

The internal mechanical energy of the inner layer modeled as an orthotropic shell has the following form [19]:

$$U_2 = 0.5[C_{11}^2(\varepsilon_x^2)^2 + 2C_{12}^2\varepsilon_x^2\varepsilon_\theta^2 + C_{22}^2(\varepsilon_\theta^2)^2] + 2G^2(\varepsilon_{x\theta}^2)^2 + 0.5[D_{11}^2(\kappa_x^2)^2 + 2D_{12}^2\kappa_x^2\kappa_\theta^2 + D_{22}^2(\kappa_\theta^2)^2] + 2D_\tau^2(\tau^2)^2$$

where C_{11}^2, C_{12}^2, and C_{22}^2 are orthotropic in-plane moduli; D_{11}^2, D_{12}^2, and D_{22}^2 are orthotropic bending and twisting moduli, and κ_x^2, κ_θ^2, and τ^2 are the components of the curvature and twist changes of the inner layer.

The constitutive relations and equilibrium equations for the two layers are derived on the basis of thermodynamic potential by varying it in terms of the strains, the wall potential, and the displacements. In the case of the axial symmetry (when there is no θ dependence of the wall characteristics), the constitutive relations for the active layer take the following form:

$$N_x^1 = C_{11}^1\varepsilon_x^1 + C_{12}^1\varepsilon_\theta^1 + f_x(\Delta\psi)$$

$$N_\theta^1 = C_{12}\varepsilon_x^1 + C_{11}\varepsilon_\theta^1 + f_\theta(\Delta\psi)$$

$$M_x^1 = D_{11}^1\kappa_x^1,\ M_\theta^1 = D_{12}^1\kappa_x^1$$

$$D = hf'_x(\Delta\psi)\varepsilon_\theta^1 + hf'_\theta(\Delta\psi)\varepsilon_\theta^1 + hG'(\Delta\psi)$$

where N_x^1 and N_θ^1 are the components of the in-plane resultant forces, M_x^1 and M_θ^1 are the components of the bending moment, and D is the electric displacement in the active layer.

We introduce the passive and active components of the strains as:

$$\varepsilon_x^1 = \varepsilon_x^p + \varepsilon_x^a,\ \varepsilon_\theta^1 = \varepsilon_\theta^p + \varepsilon_\theta^a$$

where

$$\vec{\varepsilon}(\varepsilon_x^p, \varepsilon_\theta^p) = [C^1]^{-1}\vec{N}(N_x^1, N_\theta^1)$$

where $[C^1]$ is the 2 × 2 matrix of the C-moduli for the active layer. These definitions mean that the passive component corresponds to the strains generated by the resultant forces under the conditions of the unchanged wall potential, and the active component corresponds to strains generated by electric potential under the conditions of the unchanged resultant forces.

For the passive layer, the constitutive relations reduce to the following system:

$$N_x^2 = C_{11}^2\varepsilon_x^2 + C_{12}^2\varepsilon_\theta^2$$

$$N_\theta^2 = C_{12}^2\varepsilon_x^2 + C_{22}^2\varepsilon_\theta^2$$

$$M_x^2 = D_{11}^2\kappa_x^2,\ M_\theta^2 = D_{12}^2\kappa_\theta^2$$

where N_x^2 and N_θ^2 are the components of the in-plane resultant forces, and M_x^2 and M_θ^2 are the components of the bending moment.

The equilibrium equations for an element of the cell wall take the form:

$$\frac{\partial N_x^1}{\partial x} + k_x(u_x^1 - u_x^2) = 0$$

$$\frac{\partial N_x^2}{\partial x} - k_x(u_x^1 - u_x^2) = 0$$

$$\frac{\partial^2 M_x^1}{\partial x^2} + \frac{N_\theta^1}{a} + k_n \frac{(w^1 - w^2)}{a} = p^1$$

$$\frac{\partial^2 M_x^2}{\partial x^2} + \frac{N_\theta^2}{a} - k_n \frac{(w^1 - w^2)}{a} = p^2$$

Here, we neglect shear effects of the fluids inside and outside the cell as well as within the extracisternal space. The effect of these fluids enters the equilibrium equations through pressure gradients p^1 and p^2 across the active and passive layers, respectively.

Results and Discussion

As an application of the proposed model, we consider the problem of the cell electrical stimulation under the conditions of the microchamber experiment [20, 21]. We assume the uniformity and axisymmetry of the stresses and strains along the cell. We consider the pillars much stiffer than other components of the wall, and this assumption results in the following equations:

$$\varepsilon_x^1 = \varepsilon_x^2 = \varepsilon_x^a$$

$$\varepsilon_\theta^1 = \varepsilon_\theta^2 = \varepsilon_\theta^a$$

We also neglect additional pressure generated inside the cell as a result of the electromotile strains, an assumption analyzed in Dallos et al. [20], Tolomeo and Steele [22], and Spector et al. [16]. Since no additional pressure under the conditions of consideration is created, there are no changes in the overall (i.e., for the whole wall) resultant forces. On the basis of the constitutive relations and equilibrium equations, we can express the components of the active force in terms of the electromotile (active) strains and elastic moduli of the wall components:

$$f_x = -(C_{11}^1 + C_{11}^2)\varepsilon_x^a - (C_{12}^1 + C_{12}^2)\varepsilon_\theta^a$$

$$f_\theta = -(C_{12}^1 + C_{12}^2)\varepsilon_x^a - (C_{22}^1 + C_{22}^2)\varepsilon_\theta^a$$

We can also determine elastic energy accumulated within the active and passive layers as a result of the electrical excitation of the cell. This energy for the two layers is determined by the following expressions:

$$U_1 = 0.5[C_{11}^1(\varepsilon_x^a)^2 + 2C_{12}^1\varepsilon_x^a\varepsilon_\theta^a + C_{11}^1(\varepsilon_\theta^a)^2]$$

$$U_2 = 0.5[C_{11}^2(\varepsilon_x^a)^2 + 2C_{12}^2\varepsilon_x^a\varepsilon_\theta^a + C_{22}^2(\varepsilon_\theta^a)^2]$$

We next find the active strains, active forces, and elastic energy generated by the cell wall as functions of the applied voltage. The active strains can be estimated directly from the data of the microchamber experiment [20, 21]. It should be emphasized that the active strains determined here on the basis of a particular experiment are universal characteristics of the outer hair cell's plasma membrane. They determine the response of the plasma membrane to the electric potential challenge under conditions of unchanged membrane forces (stresses). The dependence of the active strains on the membrane potential is illustrated in figure 2. The two components have opposite signs, and the absolute value of the circumferential component is about 3.5 times greater than that of the longitudinal one. The saturation is clear for the direction of the cell hyperpolarization. It is less observable for the cell depolarization direction.

The active force is a characteristic of the outer hair cell behavior that is crucial for the active processes in the cochlea. The derived equations for the components of the active force show that the stiffness of both layers, active and passive, contributes to the active force. There are different interpretations of experimental data in terms of the plasma membrane's stiffness relative to the stiffness of the rest of the wall. An important conclusion that can be derived on the basis of our expressions for the active force is that there is a component of the active force independent of the passive properties of the plasma membrane. This component is determined by the active strains and the stiffness of the passive layer, and it can be generated by the wall with a very low relative stiffness of the plasma membrane (C^1 stiffness moduli are much smaller than C^2 stiffness moduli).

We use the previously estimated overall properties of the cell wall [12, 15] and the data from the microchamber experiment to find the voltage dependence for the components of the active forces (fig. 3). The two components have opposite signs, and the circumferential component is about 2 times greater in absolute value. The nonlinearity is much more pronounced in the hyperpolarization range. The slope of the longitudinal component at the point of the resting potential determines the coefficient of the active force production per unit of the membrane potential change. In comparison to independently obtained experimental data, our estimate is about 30% lower than the results [23] obtained in the whole cochlea. The present estimate is about 1.3 and 1.8 times, respectively, greater than the measurements [21, 24] in an isolated cell. Our result is close to the maximal value and about 4 times greater than the mean value of the active force currently estimated [25].

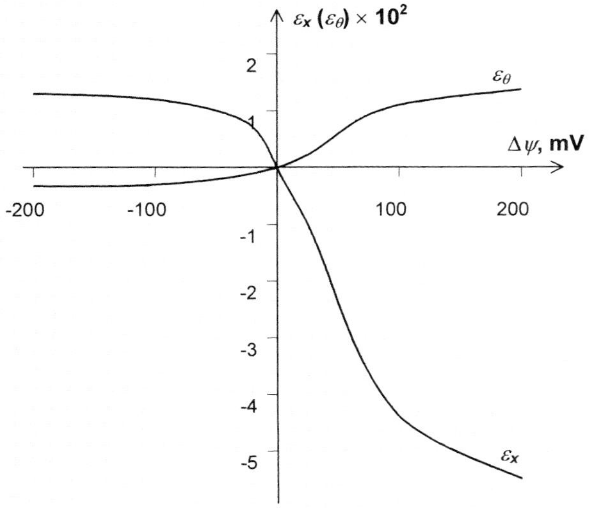

Fig. 2. Two components of the active strain generated within the active layer (plasma membrane) versus the membrane potential (x-direction along the cell, θ-direction around the cell).

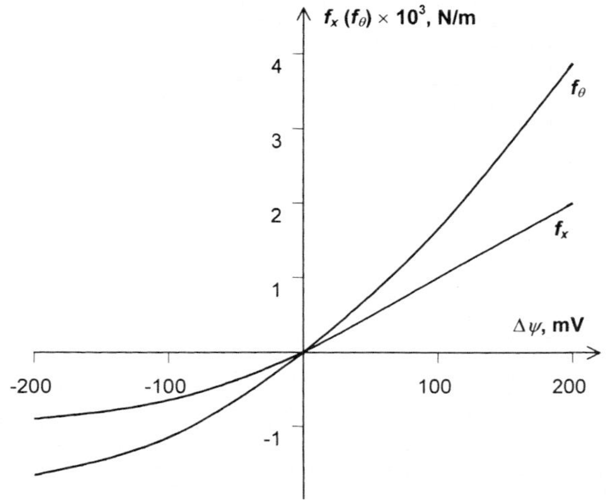

Fig. 3. Two components of the active force generated by the cell wall versus the membrane potential.

We also plot the voltage dependence of mechanical energy accumulated in the active and passive layers. This characteristic for two layers is determined by functions U_1 and U_2. There are no reliable data on the C^1 and C^2 moduli that would allow us to plot the quantitative values of U_1 and U_2. To show a qualitative dependence of mechanical energy stored in two layers on the membrane voltage, we use dimensionless functions given by the following equations:

$$U_1^* = \frac{U_1}{0.5C_{11}^1(\varepsilon_x^-)^2},\quad U_2^* = \frac{U_2}{0.5C_{11}^2(\varepsilon_x^-)^2}$$

Here, ε_x^- denotes the limiting value of the x-component of the active strain corresponding to the extreme hyperpolarization of the wall [substituted from 20]. The plasma membrane is low compressible because of the presence of a lipid bilayer. This means that the C_{12}^1 modulus is close to the C_{11}^1 modulus. We assume them equal, and this assumption completely specifies elastic energy U_1^* as a function of the active strains (the membrane potential). We need additional assumptions to specify elastic energy U_2^*. The ratio C_{22}^2/C_{11}^2 determines anisotropy of the passive layer. In this composite layer, the cytoskeleton is anisotropic and the subsurface cisternae can be considered isotropic. This means that anisotropy of the whole passive layer is lower than that for the cytoskeleton. The above ratio of two moduli for isolated cytoskeleton has been measured [26]. It was estimated to be close to 6. We use this estimate as an upper bound of the C_{22}^2/C_{11}^2 ratio for the whole passive layer. The second ratio, C_{12}^2/C_{11}^2, entering the expression of elastic energy U_2^* has the following upper bound [13]:

$$\frac{C_{12}^2}{C_{11}^2} < \sqrt{\frac{C_{22}^2}{C_{11}^2}}$$

Based on those bounds, we chose ranges for the ratios of elastic moduli entering U_2^*. In figures 4 and 5 we present a set of graphs giving the voltage dependence of elastic energy U_2^* for several values of the ratios of elastic moduli. These values belong to the above-discussed ranges. The graph for the voltage dependence of elastic energy U_1^* is also presented in figure 5. All graphs show similar behavior. For the chosen reference value –70 mV, hyperpolarization is accompanied by much greater mechanical energy than depolarization corresponding to the same magnitude of the potential change. It results in the strong asymmetry with respect to the reference point of both functions U_1^* and U_2^*. Magnitude of mechanical energy for both

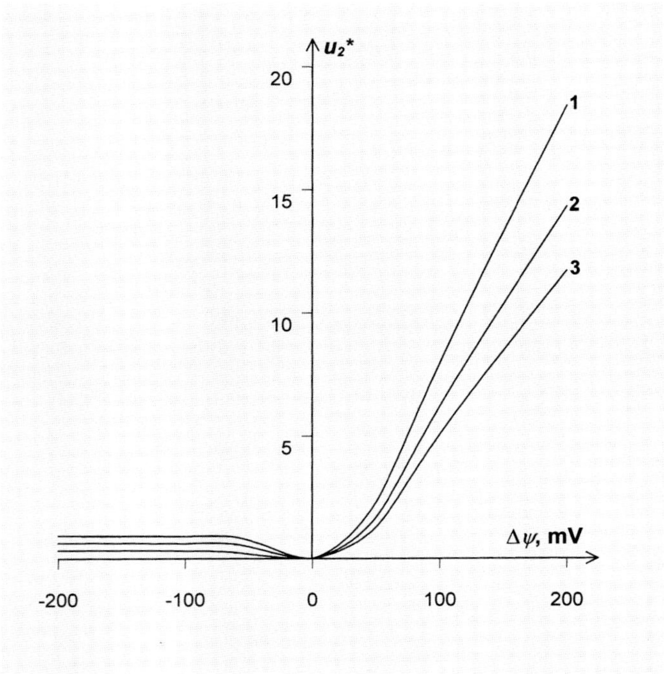

Fig. 4. Mechanical energy U_2^* stored in the passive layer for different ratios of its elastic moduli versus the membrane potential (C_{22}^2/C_{11}^2 = 3 and 1, 2, and 3 correspond, respectively, to C_{12}^2/C_{11}^2 = 1, 1.3, and 1.5).

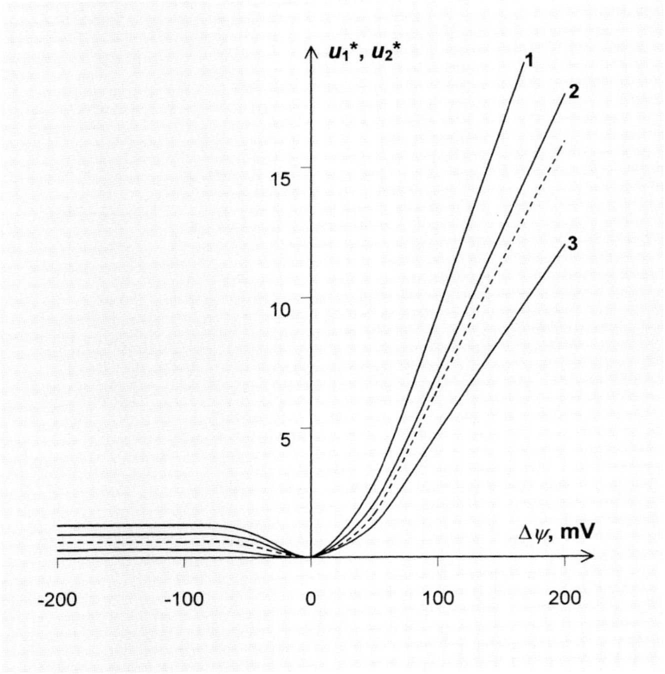

Fig. 5. Mechanical energy U_2^* stored in the passive layer for different ratios of its elastic moduli (C_{22}^2/C_{11}^2 = 5 and 1, 2, and 3 correspond, respectively, to C_{12}^2/C_{11}^2 = 1, 1.4, and 1.8); also mechanical energy U_1^* stored in the active layer versus the membrane potential (dotted line).

layers saturates for extreme hyperpolarization of the membrane. This behavior is similar to that for the absolute values of the active force and active strain.

The proposed approach is a basis for more detailed molecular-level models of outer hair cell mechanics and electromotility [e.g., 27] both for normal and pathological conditions. It can be used for a rational exploration of the experimental data to physiological conditions for which direct measurements have not been available. This approach can be also used for advanced models of the organ of Corti and the whole cochlea.

References

1 Liberman MC: Chronic ultrastructural changes in acoustic trauma: Serial-section reconstruction of stereocilia and cuticular plates. Hear Res 1987;26:65–88.
2 Chan E, Suneson A, Ulfendahl M: Acoustic trauma causes reversible stiffness changes in auditory sensory cells. Neuroscience 1998;83:961–968.
3 Shehata WE, Brownell WE, Dieler R: Effects of salicylate on shape, electromotility and membrane characteristics of isolated outer hair cells from the guinea pig cochlea. Acta Otolaryngol (Stockh) 1991;11:707–718.
4 Russell IJ, Schauz C: Salicylate ototoxicity: Effects on the stiffness and electromotility of outer hair cells isolated from the guinea pig cochlea. Aud Neurosci 1995;1:309–320.
5 Lue AJC, Weng TX, Spector AA, Popel AS, Brownell WE: Salicylate-induced changes of outer hair cell lateral wall stiffness; in Popelka GR (ed): Abstr 19th Annual ARO Research Meeting, Des Moines 1996, p 62.
6 Dieler R, Shehata-Dieler WE, Brownell WE: Concomitant salicylate-induced alterations of outer hair cell subsurface cisternae and electromotility. J Neurocytol 1991;20:637–653.
7 Hallworth R: Modulation of OHC force generation and stiffness by agents known to affect hearing; in Lewis GR, Long GR, Lyon RF, Narins PM, Steele CR, Hecht-Poinar E (eds): Diversity in Auditory Mechanics. Singapore, World Scientific, 1997, pp 524–530.
8 Tunstall MJ, Gale JE, Ashmore JF: Action of salicylate on membrane capacitance of outer hair cells from the guinea-pig cochlea. J Physiol 1995;485:739–752.
9 Karlsson KK, Flock Å: Quinine causes isolated outer hair cells to change length. Neurosci Lett 1990;116:101–105.

10 Schuknecht HF: Pathology of the Ear, ed 2. Philadelphia, Lea & Febiger, 1993.
11 Schulte BA, Schmiedt RA: Lateral wall Na, K-ATPase and endocochlear potentials decline with age in quiet-reared gerbils. Hear Res 1992; 61:35–46.
12 Spector AA: A nonlinear electroelastic model of the cochlear outer hair cell; in Gonçalves PB, Jasiuk I, Pamplona D, Steele CR, Weber HI, Bevilacqua L (eds): Applied Mechanics in the Americas. Rio de Janeiro, American Academy of Mechanics, 1999, vol 6, pp 19–22.
13 Spector AA, Brownell WE, Popel AS: Elastic properties of the composite outer hair cell wall. Ann Biomed Eng 1998;26:157–165.
14 Kalinec F, Holley MC, Iwasa KH, Lim DJ, Kachar B: A membrane-based force generation mechanism in auditory sensory cells. Proc Natl Acad Sci USA 1992;89:8671–8675.
15 Spector AA, Brownell WE, Popel AS: Estimation of elastic moduli and bending stiffness of the anisotropic outer hair cell wall. J Acoust Soc Am 1998;103:1007–1011.
16 Spector AA, Brownell WE, Popel AS: Nonlinear active force generation by cochlear outer hair cell. J Acoust Soc Am 1999;105:2414–2420.
17 Kakehata S, Santos-Sacchi J: Membrane tension directly shifts voltage dependence of outer hair cell motility and associated gating charge. Biophys J 1995;68:2190–2197.
18 Gale JE, Ashmore JF: Charge displacement induced by rapid stretch in the basolateral membrane of the guinea-pig outer hair cell. Proc R Soc Lond B 1994;255:243–249.
19 Niordson FI: Shell Theory. Amsterdam, North-Holland, 1985.
20 Dallos P, Hallworth R, Evans BN: Theory of electrically driven shape changes of cochlear outer hair cells. J Neurophysiol 1993;70:299–323.
21 Hallworth R, Evans BN, Dallos P: The location and mechanism of electromotility in guinea pig outer hair cell. J Neurophysiol 1993;70:549–558.
22 Tolomeo JA, Steele CR: Orthotropic piezoelectric properties of cochlear outer hair cell wall. J Acoust Soc Am 1995;97:3006–3011.
23 Xue S, Mountain DC, Hubbard AE: Direct measurement of electrically-evoked basilar membrane motion; in Duifhuis H, Horst JW, van Dijk P, van Netten SM (eds): Biophysics of Hair Cell Sensory Systems. Singapore, World Scientific, 1993, pp 361–368.
24 Iwasa KH, Adachi M: Force generation in the outer hair cell of the cochlea. Biophys J 1997; 73:546–555.
25 Frank G, Hemmert W, Gummer AW: Limiting dynamics of high-frequency electromechanical transduction of outer hair cells. Proc Natl Acad Sci USA 1999;96:4420–4425.
26 Tolomeo JA, Steele CR, Holley MC: Mechanical properties of the lateral cortex of mammalian auditory outer hair cells. Biophys J 1996;71: 421–429.
27 Spector AA, Ameen M, Charalambides PG, Popel AS: Mechanical properties of the outer hair cell cytoskeleton: Simulation of the microstructure and molecular organization; in Goel VK et al (ed): Summer Bioengineering Conference. New York, ASME, 1999, pp 325–326.

ORL
ORL 1999;61:294–304

A Physiological Ear Model for the Emulation of Masking

Frank Baumgarte

Institut für Theoretische Nachrichtentechnik und Informationsverarbeitung, Universität Hannover, Germany

Key Words

Audio coding · Auditory masking · Auditory model · Cochlear amplifier · Cochlear model · Data compression · Dynamic compression · Distortion products · Loudness modeling · Two-tone suppression

Abstract

Auditory masking is exploited in technical audio systems for transmission and storage to improve the perceived audio quality. In this respect, perception models are necessary for a masked threshold prediction to quantify the threshold of audibility for a given signal or distortion. The presented ear model emulates those parts of the auditory sound processing which are relevant to masking. The physiological modeling approach is not limited to simple masker-test-signal configurations as usually employed in psychoacoustical measurements, but it is valid for complex signals as well, which is desired in the aforementioned applications. The ear model includes a nonlinear active cochlear model which emulates the basic mechanisms effective in masking: excitation and suppression. Nonlinear mechanical amplification by means of the outer hair cells plays a crucial role in proper modeling of these effects. In addition to physiological measurements at the mechanical level of sound processing in the cochlea, classical masking patterns and nonlinear masking effects are demonstrated by the ear model.

Introduction

The investigation of masking effects in psychoacoustics represents an appropriate method for deriving information about sound processing properties of the human auditory system. Results from these investigations are important as well for quantitative modeling of masking effects employed in technical applications like audio data compression or perceptual audio quality assessment. In the past, models for auditory masking were widely based solely on psychoacoustical masked threshold measurements, so that known physiological properties of sound processing were not considered explicitly.

In psychoacoustical listening tests masked thresholds are measured for combinations of simple masker and test signals like pure tones or narrow-band noise. They are determined by a given probability, e.g. 50% of test signal audibility in the presence of the masker. Masking primarily depends on the masker signal characteristics and shows

KARGER

Fax + 41 61 306 12 34
E-Mail karger@karger.ch
www.karger.com

© 1999 S. Karger AG, Basel
0301–1569/99/0615–0294$17.50/0

Accessible online at:
http://BioMedNet.com/karger

Frank Baumgarte
Institut für Theoretische Nachrichtentechnik und Informationsverarbeitung
Appelstrasse 9A, D–30167 Hannover (Germany)
Tel. +49 511 762 5047, Fax +49 511 762 5052
E-Mail baumgart@tnt.uni-hannover.de

highly nonlinear properties. Technical applications require a masked threshold prediction by a perception model for very complex signals, e.g. speech or music. This prediction is usually based on an extrapolation from measurements for simple masker-test-signal configurations. However, an extrapolation using a simple superposition is generally not appropriate since the highly nonlinear properties of auditory sound processing have significant effects on masking.

The physiological modeling approach accounts for these nonlinearities and is valid for arbitrary complex signals. Furthermore, the ear model is founded on both physiological and psychoacoustical measurements, which is a reasonable approach to simulate masking of arbitrary complex signals beyond the scope of psychoacoustical masking experiments.

The ear model is primarily designed for applications in data compression realized by audio coding schemes. Nevertheless, due to the general modeling approach, it provides physiological and psychoacoustical simulation results which are relevant to basic auditory research. A more detailed description of the ear model than given in this paper is available [1–3].

The next section reviews basic physiological masking properties considered by the ear model. A description of the physiological ear model structure follows, complemented by results from physiological and psychoacoustical simulations in comparison to measurements. Main findings and conclusions are finally summarized.

Fundamentals of Auditory Physiology

The auditory system is functionally subdivided into a peripheral and a central part. The boundary is assumed to be located at the initial level of neural activity, the generation of action potentials in individual fibers of the auditory nerve by the inner hair cells (IHCs). This boundary differentiates between the two basic sound signal representations: the mechanical representation in the periphery and the electrical representation in the central auditory system. The physiological properties of the periphery are widely known, although underlying details are still subject to debate. In contrast, sound processing in the central auditory system is far from being known in all physiological processes involved. This is why psychoacoustical measurements have to be consulted to derive input-output functions of this part. A description of the central auditory system is omitted here since the details are not required to understand the ear model.

The cochlea of the inner ear comprises the sound processing and transducing organ which provides a signal analysis resulting in a spectro-temporal activity pattern. The coiled, fluid-filled cochlea is divided lengthwise by the cochlear partition in two mechanically effective chambers. This partition contains the organ of Corti attached to the basilar membrane (BM) as the major parts shown in figure 1. The width and compliance of the BM increase with the distance from the oval window at the cochlear entrance. Vibrations of the oval window create pressure variations in the fluid entailing transverse vibrations of the cochlear partition. For a single frequency stimulation a traveling wave propagates from the oval window towards the apex with increasing transverse BM displacement which builds up to a maximum at a fixed place and shows a rapid decline thereafter which will be illustrated later by simulation results. The longitudinal BM location of the maximum shifts with higher signal frequency towards the oval window. In this way, the envelope of the transverse BM velocity represents the input signal spectral analysis which converts frequency to place information.

The organ of Corti transduces the cochlear partition velocity into action potentials on the auditory nerve by means of the IHCs, the acoustical sensory cells. In addition to the place of activity, the amount of activity in terms of the number of action potentials per time and the temporal envelope and fine structure of the impulse patterns makes up the coded signal information in each fiber of the auditory nerve.

The outer hair cells (OHCs) support the adaptation of the input signal dynamic range to the limitations of the IHCs. Today it is generally accepted that small BM vibrations are mechanically amplified by the OHCs [4]. The OHC amplification behaves nonlinearly since it saturates at medium sound levels so that it has negligible effect at high levels. Amplification factors in the order of 1,000 are observed in mammals at low sound levels [5, 6]. The nonlinear mechanical amplification provides the common explanation for many nonlinear effects in hearing and especially in masking.

Masking and Loudness

Masked thresholds determined in psychoacoustical experiments are the reference data to be approximated by the physiological ear model proposed here. In simple masking experiments subjects are exposed with a masker signal of constant spectral envelope and finite duration. They are instructed to detect the test signal in presence of

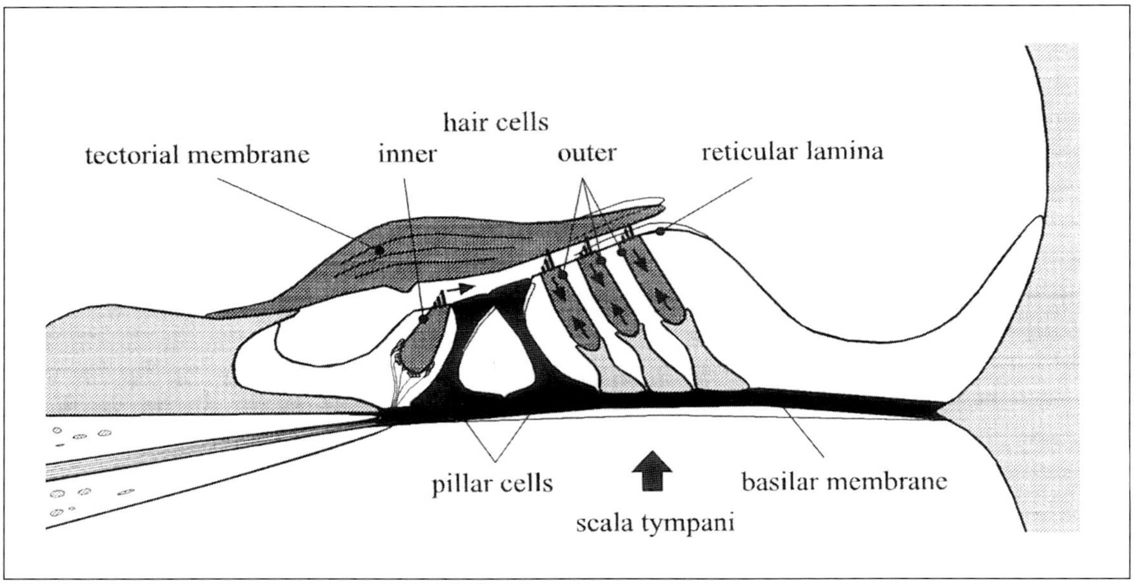

Fig. 1. Cross-section of cochlear partition with tectorial membrane, basilar membrane (BM), and organ of Corti comprising inner (IHCs) and outer hair cells (OHCs) as major parts. A transverse displacement (large arrow) of the BM results in a deflection of the hair cell stereociliae. The OHCs mechanically amplify this stimulation signal due to an active length change. The IHCs transduce the mechanical stimulation into a neural signal representation.

the masker, e.g. a pure tone presented at a certain temporal position relative to the masker. Usually, several signal intervals are presented allowing a direct comparison between the sole masker and the masker with superimposed test signal. The test signal level at the threshold of audibility is the masked threshold for the chosen combination of masker and test signal. Spectral representations of masked thresholds are advantageously scaled and explored using critical-band rates in Bark units [7]. The critical-band-rate scale reflects the resonance frequency distribution along the BM assigning the local BM resonance frequencies to a spatially uniform Bark scale.

Loudness quantifies the sensation of sound intensity. Total loudness of sound is represented by a single value which can be time-varying. Loudness may also be spectrally decomposed into critical bands resulting in a specific loudness function over a critical-band-rate scale. Loudness is taken into consideration because masked thresholds can be interpreted as just-noticeable changes in specific loudness. This idea is a fundamental assumption for the modeling approach which is described later. In the aforementioned simple masking experiment the masked threshold can thus be explained by the change in specific loudness caused by the superimposed test signal. This change is detectable according to the model of just-noticeable changes [8] if it exceeds a presumed threshold value. A comprehensive description of procedures and results of masking and loudness measurements is given in Zwicker and Fastl [7].

Physiological Ear Model

As outlined in the block diagram of figure 2, the ear model reflects the processing structure of the auditory system. The peripheral ear is represented by a model of the outer and middle ear (OME) which is connected to the cochlear model consisting of a model of cochlear hydromechanics (HM), OHC models, and IHC models. The neural processing (NP) models are fed by the output of the IHC models. The masked threshold for a test signal in the presence of a masker is generated iteratively by first calculating the specific loudness of the sole masker, and in a second step for the masker with superimposed test signal. The change in specific loudness caused by the test signal is assessed afterwards by the NP models in order to decide whether a signal change is audible and to adjust the test signal level accordingly for the next iteration step. The iteration continues until the test signal level is adjusted sufficiently close to the masked threshold level.

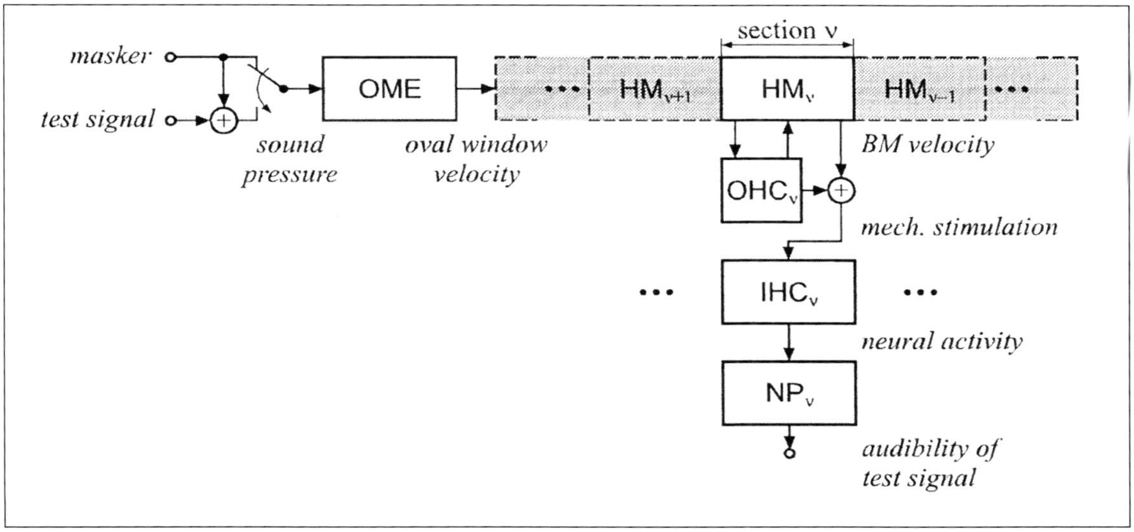

Fig. 2. Block diagram of the physiological ear model with following model parts: outer and middle ear model (OME), cochlear hydromechanics (HM_ν), outer hair cell (OHC_ν), inner hair cell (IHC_ν), and neural processing (NP_ν). Only one section is shown – the other sections have identical structure.

The model of the peripheral ear is specified as electrical network using the correspondence of voltages and currents in electrical systems to associated velocities and forces in acoustical or mechanical systems respectively. It is simulated in the time domain by wave digital filters [9] preserving the stability properties of the corresponding analog circuit in the digital domain. This simulation technique is a computationally efficient method in cochlear modeling [10].

The OME model is desigend as a linear prefilter for the incoming sound signal. The magnitude frequency response shows increased damping at a rate of 6 dB/octave for decreasing frequencies below 1 kHz and a resonance at 3 kHz. Thus it considers the low-frequency damping of the middle ear and the first ear-canal resonance. The acoustics of the outer and middle ear is not considered for frequencies higher than 3 kHz because numerous resonances occur in this range inside the ear canal which deviate interindividually. Hence, as an average for high frequencies a constant magnitude response is assumed (cf. fig. 3).

The velocity of the oval window provided by the OME model as corresponding voltage u_{OW} is applied at the entrance of the cochlear model. A model of the passive cochlear hydromechanics can be derived from the dimensions and material properties of the inner ear. If all micromechanical elements of the cochlear partition are assumed to move with the same transverse velocity, and with further reasonable simplifications, a one-dimensional mechanical model can be formulated [11]. This mechanical model is transformed into a dual electrical network with discrete elements. The cochlear model proposed by Zwicker and Peisl [12, 13] extends this passive system by active OHC models. This proposed model served as base for the extended cochlear model as part of the ear model presented here. Both cochlear models make

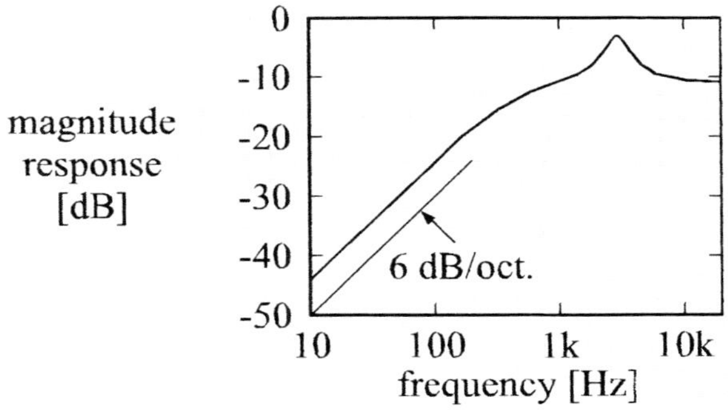

Fig. 3. Magnitude response of the outer and middle ear model loaded by the input impedance of the subsequent model parts.

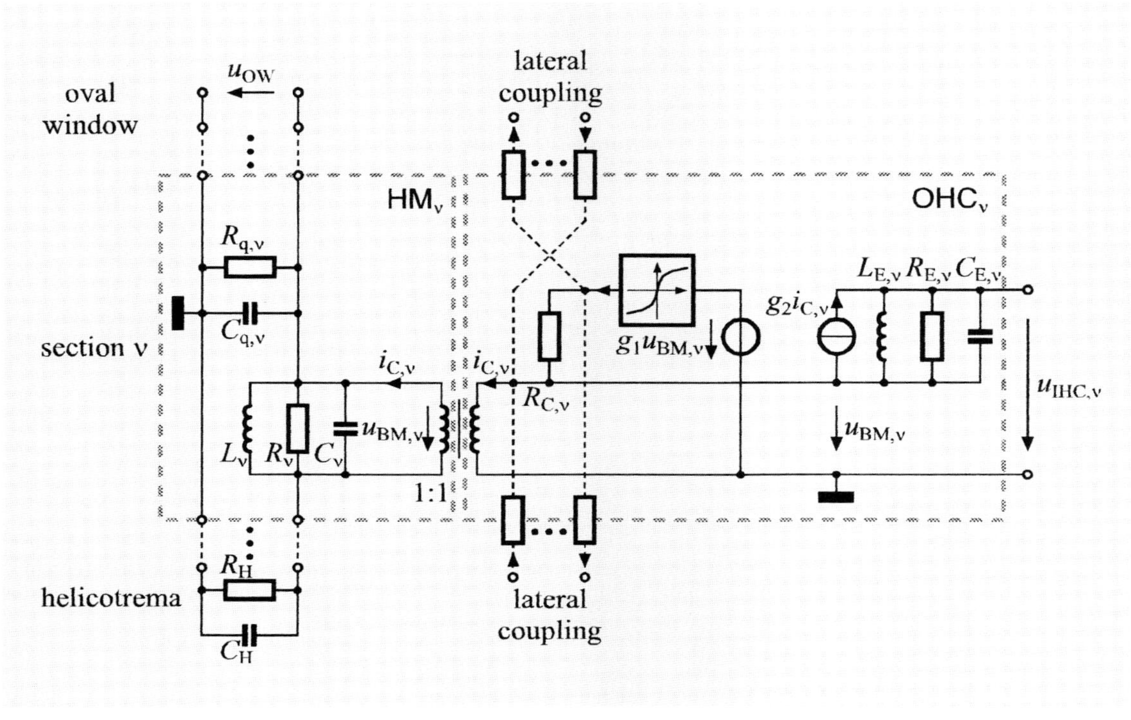

Fig. 4. Cochlear model without inner hair cell model. The ν-th section is shown consisting of the model parts of the hydromechanics (HM_ν) complemented by the outer hair cell (OHC_ν) model. The remaining sections have identical structure. Only a part of the coupling resistances between neighboring sections is shown, denoted with 'lateral coupling'.

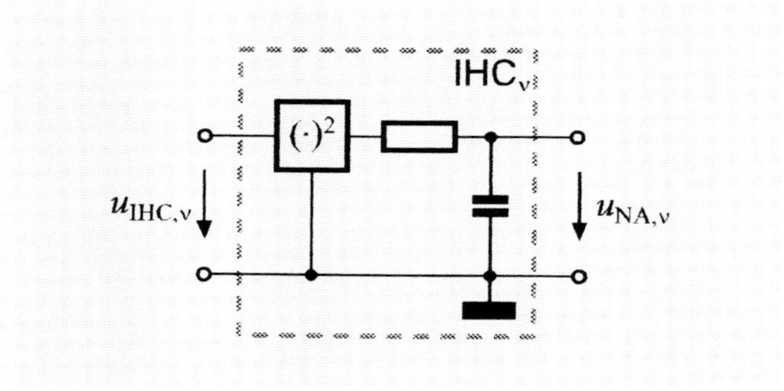

Fig. 5. Electrical network model of the inner hair cell.

use of wave digital filters which allow the simulation of otoacoustic emissions (OAE). One section of the extended cochlear model consists of the HM model part and the OHC model as shown in figure 4. The HM model emulates the hydromechanics of the cochlear duct and the cochlear partition corresponding to the passive model [11]. Each section of the HM model corresponds to one of the slices created by dividing the unrolled cochlear duct into parts of equal length. A total number of 241 sections was used to represent the cochlea from oval window to helicotrema at the cochlear apex. Each model section contains a parallel resonance circuit representing the local BM resonance which determines the so-called 'characteristic frequency' (CF). The additional capacitor $C_{q,\nu}$ and resistance $R_{\nu,b}$ in each section accounts for the damping and longitudinal mechanical coupling by the fluid. The voltage u_{BM} represents the transverse BM velocity which is amplified by g_1 in the OHC model inside a feedback loop with a nonlinear characteristic resulting in a continuously growing saturation for increasing level. At low signal levels the nonlinearity causes a high u_{BM} gain for frequencies near the section resonance in comparison to the passive system. In addition, the antisymmetric characteristic produces odd order distortions. A second amplification stage is added to achieve a resulting maximum

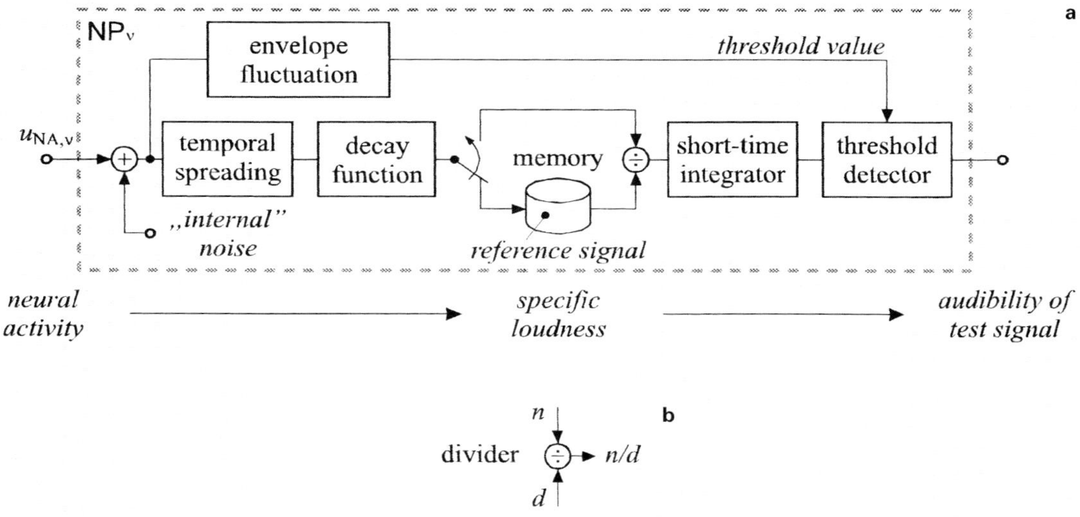

Fig. 6a, b. Block diagram of neural processing (NP) model in one section (**a**). The masked threshold is derived by first generating the specific loudness of the reference signal (masker) which is stored in the memory. In subsequent iteration steps the test signal level is adjusted so that the specific loudness change due to the test signal superposition is at the internal threshold value. Divider symbol (**b**).

amplification of approximately 60 dB at the output of each section which approximates values found in BM measurements from mammals [5, 6]. The second stage amplifies the feedback current i_f by g_2. The current source is loaded by a parallel resonance circuit identical to the circuit in the HM model of the same section. Both impedances have identical frequency dependencies which ensures that also both associated voltages have the same frequency dependence and are in phase. In this network structure the additional stage is necessary to maintain stability for such a high amplification, since the amplifier in the feedback loop preserves stability up to approximately 40 dB gain. The extension by the second amplification stage is the only modification compared to the cochlear model structure given in Zwicker and Peisl [12] and Peisl [13]. Neighboring OHC models are coupled via resistors with increasing resistances for increasing section distances. Each section is coupled with 16 sections to either side. However, this is only shown for the directly neighboring sections in figure 4.

The second amplification stage generates the stimulation signal u_{IHC} for the IHC model in each section. The IHC model consists of a square function and a low-pass filter as shown in figure 5. These two elements approximate the half-wave rectification and the low-pass characteristic as basic properties of the IHCs. Different types of nerve fibers connected to an IHC operate at different input signal levels and show a limited dynamic range [15]. These properties are not considered in detail, it is rather assumed that the full dynamic range is transmitted by the different auditory nerve fibers without limiting or compression. The IHC model integrates a square function to account for psychoacoustical measurements which show that the central auditory system behaves approximately linear with respect to sound intensity [14]. From a physiological viewpoint, however, the realization of this square function may be located in a higher processing stage of the auditory system.

The IHC model output signals represent the degree of neural activity of the auditory nerve fibers connected to the IHCs at the BM location corresponding to the model section. Neural activity can be interpreted as the spatial and short-term averaged number of action potentials per time interval.

The physiological processes in the auditory pathways and cortex are not completely understood, so that a psychoacoustical modeling approach is assumed to be appropriate for the central auditory system. A simplified block diagram of the NP model is given in figure 6, where each block accounts for the proper modeling of a specific masking effect.

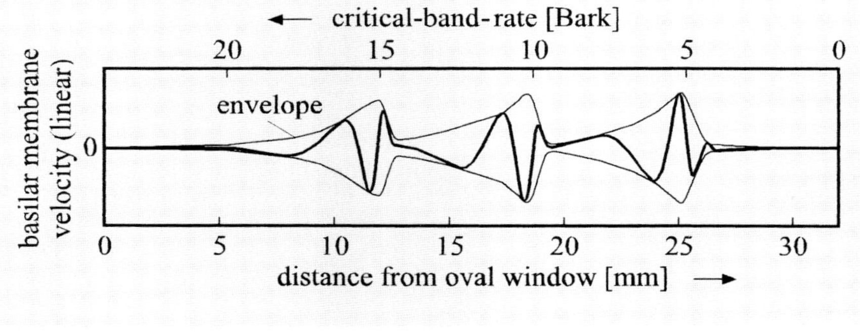

Fig. 7. BM velocity calculated for three superimposed sinusoids with 60 dB SPL and critical-band-rates of 5, 10, and 15 Bark. The traveling wave propagates from left to right with the local velocity maxima and minima in coincidence with the envelope. The critical-band-rate scale is linearly related to the BM position and corresponds to the local characteristic frequency (CF).

Internal noise is added to the input neural activity signal to limit the audibility of signals to the range above threshold in quiet. A temporal spread function is applied afterwards to account for the limited masked threshold rise time in premasking. The temporal spread may be attributed to different signal propagation times on the auditory pathways. A decay function, which is adapted to the masker level and duration, models the most important properties of postmasking and may be attributed to the recovery time of nerve cells after stimulation, including the IHC synapse. The output signal at this stage is assumed to represent specific loudness [7]. A short-time integrator, realized as first-order low-pass filter, is applied to the specific loudness change which is caused by a superimposed test signal and calculated as the specific loudness ratio of the masker plus test signal and the sole masker (reference). The short-time integration reflects the dependency of masking on test signal duration, e.g. a brief test signal is less audible than a test signal of the same level and longer duration. The threshold detector is fed by the integrator output. Each time its input value exceeds the threshold, the change caused by the test signal is assumed to be audible. Normally the change detection is independently applied in each section of the model. The threshold value in each section is adapted according to the envelope fluctuation of the nerual activity signal with internal noise added. The adaptation is necessary for the consideration of the different masking effectivity of e.g. Gaussian noise with high envelope fluctuation versus a pure tone without fluctuation.

The ear model is implemented in 'C'. Processing of an audio signal sampled at 100 kHz (for one iteration) is slower by a factor of 40 than real-time, using a PC operating at 400 MHz.

Physiological Modeling Results

The simulated transverse BM velocity is shown in figure 7 as traveling wave caused by three superimposed sinusoids. The wave envelope marks the values of the velocity maxima and minima when they propagate from oval window towards the helicotrema. The envelope shape shows three maxima, with CFs corresponding to the sinusoid frequencies, and basically depicts the selectivity of the frequency analysis filters. Each resonance location shows the typical slowly growing wave envelope before the resonance location is reached and a fast decline thereafter. Obviously, at the resonance location of the 10-Bark sinusoid, the 5-Bark sinusoid still produces significant BM motion, while the 15-Bark sinusoid has no influence at that location. This consideration illustrates why a test signal is more effectively masked by masker frequencies below than above the test signal.

Results for the IHC stimulation along the BM, which is equivalently scaled using critical-band rates, are outlined in figure 8 for 1-kHz pure tones with different sound pressure levels (SPs). The apparent features of the stimulation patterns are the dynamic compression around the CF of 1 kHz (8.5 Bark), which disappears at higher CFs, and the reduced upper slope steepness at high SPLs. BM-input/output functions are derived at the BM position where the CF is equal to the signal frequency. This function shows the dynamic level compression caused by the OHC amplification, as illustrated in figure 9. The BM-input/output function provides a compression of the dynamic range from 0 to 100 dB SPL into an IHC stimulation range spanning only 45 dB with a minimum steepness of 0.27 dB/dB at 50 dB SPL. These simulation results are in accordance with measurements from animals [5, 6].

Suppression of a test signal can be demonstrated at the mechanical level of sound processing in the cochlea. The

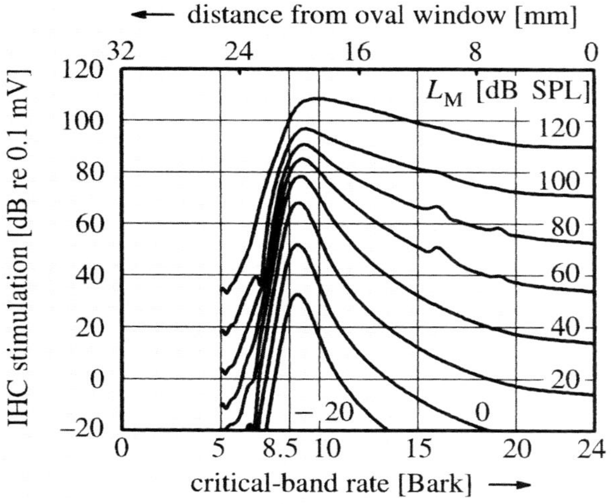

Fig. 8. IHC stimulation level at the input of the IHC model in all sections plotted on a critical-band-rate scale. A 1-kHz (8.5-Bark) sinusoid with a level of L_M is applied to the oval window HM model input.

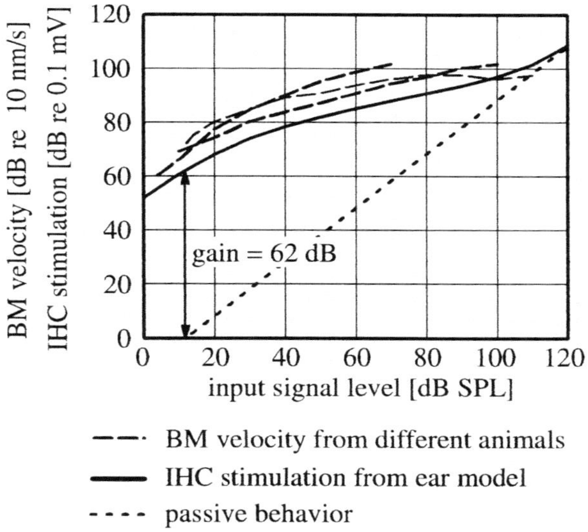

Fig. 9. Level-dependent IHC stimulation at the BM resonance location of a 1-kHz sinusoid in comparison to BM velocity measurements of different animals [6].

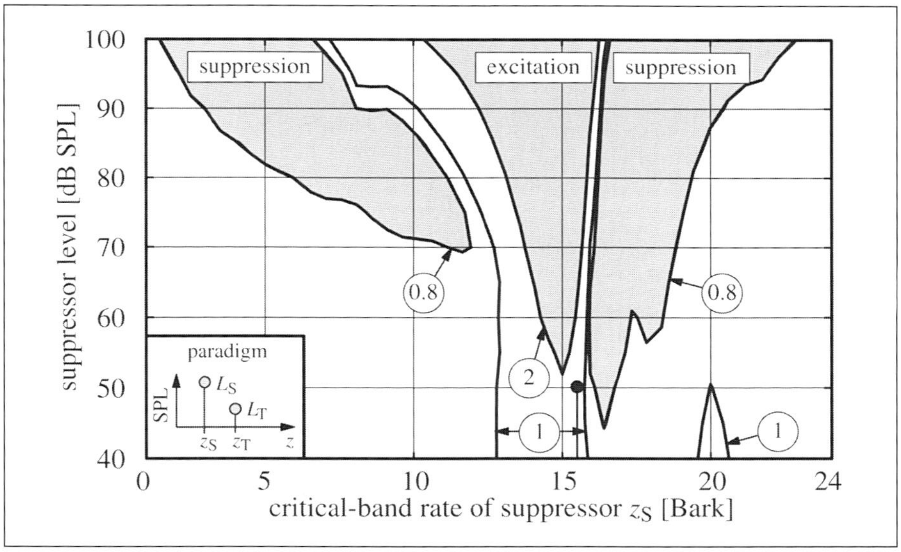

Fig. 10. Suppression tuning curves for a test tone at 3 kHz (15.7 Bark) and L_T = 50 dB SPL. Solid lines depict the contours of constant test tone suppression indicated by the encircled factors. A factor of 0.8 is equal to a suppression of 20%.

vibration amplitude of the cochlear partition caused by a sole test signal is reduced by a simultaneously superimposed suppressor signal within bounded areas in the suppressor frequency-level plane. Apart from BM vibration measurements, this phenomenon is observed in the mean firing rates of auditory nerve fibers [16]. Suppression can be explained in terms of the ear model by the saturation of the OHC amplification since a reduced test signal amplification results from those model sections where the amplifier is driven into partial saturation by the suppressor signal. Figure 10 shows simulation results for a fixed test tone at 3 kHz and 50 dB SPL. The change of the IHC

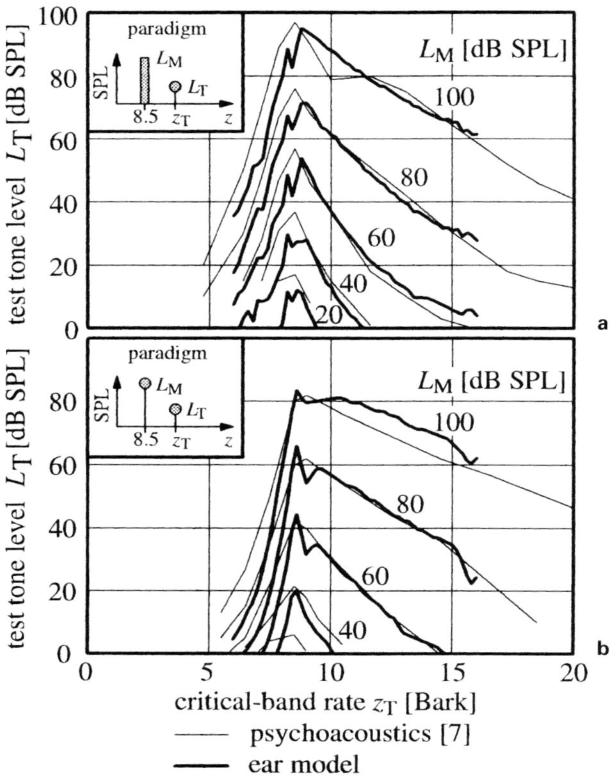

Fig. 11. Masked thresholds for a pure tone masked by narrow-band noise (**a**) or a pure tone (**b**) at 1 kHz.

stimulation signal at the corresponding resonance location is determined for different suppressor tone frequencies and levels so that a contour plot with lines of equal stimulation change can be derived. Suppression areas are defined by a stimulation reduction of more than 20%, which occur for suppressor frequencies below and above the test tone. Additionally, the excitation area where the IHC stimulation is increased by more than a factor of 2 is indicated which corresponds to measured so-called mechanical or neural 'tuning curves'. These results reflect known properties of tuning and suppression derived from measurements. Suppression of a test signal produces increased masking since the reduced vibration amplitude is less detectable in the central auditory system. Excitation results in increased masking as well because with increasing suppressor excitation the relative excitation change caused by a superimposed test signal decreases.

Psychoacoustical Modeling Results

Evaluations of the ear model using an extensive base of psychoacoustical data for different temporal and spectral masking effects have been published [2, 3]. Since most properties of simultaneous spectral masking can be traced back to a cochlear origin, the fundamental results from the simulations will be presented in the following. The classical masking patterns obtained from a narrow-band Gaussian noise or pure-tone masker and a pure test tone are shown in figure 11 for different masker levels. Simulation results are given in comparison to psychoacoustical measurements. In accordance with the asymmetrical slope steepness of the traveling-wave envelope (cf. fig. 7), the masked thresholds show a steep rise when the increased test tone frequency approaches the masker frequency and a slow decline beyond. The nonlinear level-dependent steepness of the shallower slope corresponds to the IHC stimulation signal properties in figure 8 and matches psychoacoustical measurements. Significantly lower masked thresholds observed from pure-tone maskers in comparison to a narrow-band noise masker with the same SPL are replicated by the model since the envelope fluctuation is used to control the internal detection threshold accordingly.

In figure 11 the evaluation of the signal change by the threshold detectors of the ear model was restricted to model sections near the resonance location of the test signal. This procedure is used to simulate a psychoacoustical experiment with subjects instructed to only detect the test tone itself in contrast to any arbitrary signal changes due to the test tone superposition (off-frequency listening). In the following experiment the different results for both detection schemes are compared. In figure 12 masked thresholds are plotted from measurements where subjects were asked to detect any audible change of the sound signal. Simulation results obtained for the same signal configuration are shown for the restricted case, as in the experiment described above, and the unrestricted threshold detection in all model sections. In this experiment, a narrow-band test signal with fixed frequency was utilized at four different center frequencies. The test-signal level was adjusted to the masked threshold for masker frequencies up to 4.5 Bark below and 2.5 Bark above the center frequency. Clearly audible distortion products at frequencies below the masker, most prominent at the cubic difference frequency $f_C = 2f_1 - f_2$ of the masker and test signal, result in significantly reduced masked thresholds of the shallower slope in the measurements using a test signal at 14.5 or 20.5 Bark. These masking patterns show a local

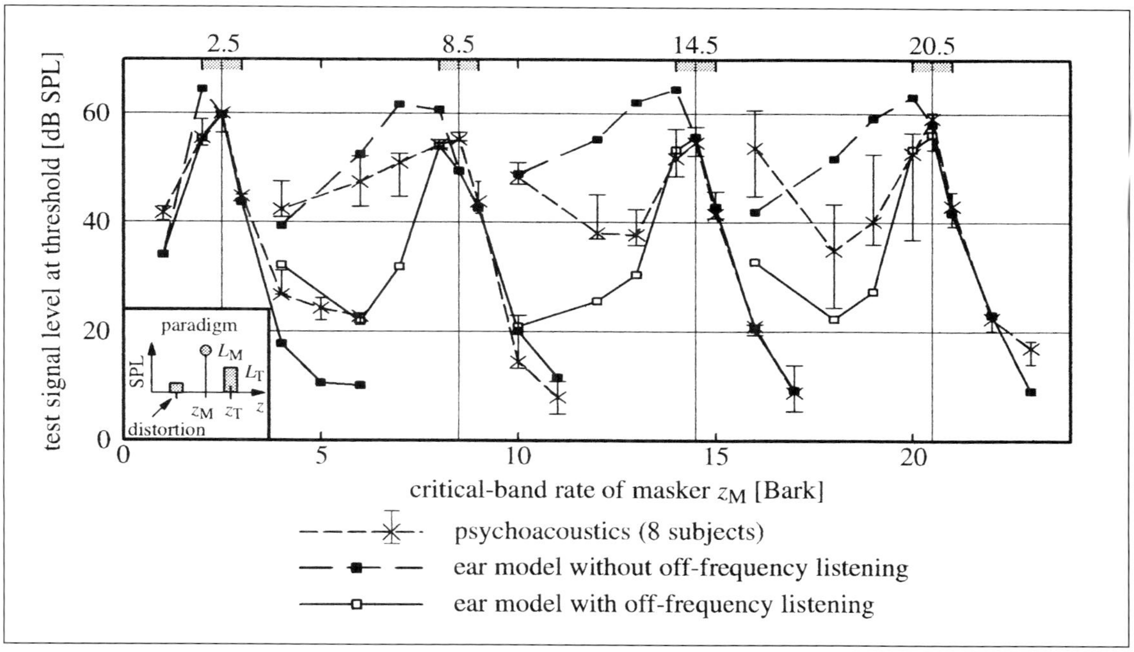

Fig. 12. Masked thresholds for critical-band noise masked by a pure tone showing psychoacoustical results with mean and interquartile ranges and modeling results. Four different critical-band wide noises were used as test signal at z_T = 2.5, 8.5, 14.5, and 20.5 Bark fixed center frequency. The masker level was constant at L_M = 80 dB SPL (M: masker, T: test signal).

minimum according to the created distortion product level and its audibility. The ear model shows the same effect since distortion products are generated by the nonlinear characteristic of the OHC amplification. However, the deviation between simulation results and measurements suggests an overestimation of the distortion product detection by the model. Nevertheless, it should be noted that the measurements also show high interindividual differences.

In summary: The presented physiological ear model emulates those parts of the human auditory system which are essential for psychoacoustical masking. Since properties of masking reflect several aspects of auditory sound processing, the ear model considers the most important physiological mechanisms effective in masking. The nonlinearity of the mechanical amplification by the outer hair cells plays a crucial role in masking and loudness perception. This nonlinearity provides a uniform modeling approach explaining many different nonlinear masking effects. For the included cochlear model a detailed micromechanical modeling is not required in this application.

In line with physiological measurements, the simulation results suggest that many features of perception and masking are already present at the mechanical level of sound processing in the cochlea. The central auditory system has merely contributions to temporal masking.

The cochlear model is based on an earlier model proposed by Zwicker and Peisl [12] and Peisl [13]. That model makes use of wave digital filters which allow the simulation of otoacoustic emissions (OAEs). The nonlinear characteristic of the OHC amplification in the model creates audible distortion products and causes dynamic compression as observed in loudness and BM vibration measurements. Physiological mechanisms of simultaneous masking consist of excitation and suppression. Both effects are also derived from the ear model in accordance with physiological measurements. The simulation results for masked thresholds are valid for simple as well as complex audio signals.

Acknowledgement

The project was supported by the Deutsche Forschungsgemeinschaft (German National Research Foundation).

References

1 Baumgarte F: Application of a physiological ear model to irrelevance reduction in audio coding. Proc 17th AES Int Conf, Signa/Italy 1999.

2 Baumgarte F: Evaluation of a physiological ear model considering masking effects relevant to audio coding. 105th AES Convention, San Francisco 1998, preprint 4789.

3 Baumgarte F: A physiological ear model for auditory masking applicable to perceptual coding. 103rd AES Convention, New York 1997, preprint 4511.

4 Spector AA, Brownell WE, Popel AS: Nonlinear active force generation by cochlear outer hair cell. J Acoust Soc Am 1999;105:2414–2420.

5 Nutall AL, Dolan DF: Steady-state sinusoidal responses of the basilar membrane in guinea pig. J Acoust Soc Am 1996;99:1556–1565.

6 Ruggero MA, Rich NC, Recio A, Narayan SS, Robles L: Basilar-membrane responses to tones at the base of the chinchilla cochlea. J Acoust Soc Am 1997;101:2151–2163.

7 Zwicker E, Fastl H: Psychoacoustics – Facts and Models, ed 2. New York, Springer, 1999.

8 Zwicker E, Feldtkeller R: Das Ohr als Nachrichtenempfänger (in German). Stuttgart, Hirzel, 1967.

9 Fettweis A: Wave digital filters: Theory and practice. Proc IEEE 1986;74:270–327.

10 Strube HW: A computational efficient basilar-membrane model. Acustica 1985;58:207–214.

11 Oetinger R, Hauser H: Ein elektrischer Kettenleiter zur Untersuchung der mechanischen Schwingungsvorgänge im Innenohr (in German). Acustica 1961;11:161–177.

12 Zwicker E, Peisl W: Cochlear preprocessing in analog models, in digital models and in human inner ear. Hear Res 1990;44:209–216.

13 Peisl W: Beschreibung aktiver nichtlinearer Effekte der peripheren Schallverarbeitung des Gehörs durch ein Rechnermodell (in German); diss, TU München 1990.

14 Plack CJ, Oxenham AJ: Basilar-membrane nonlinearity and the growth of forward masking. J Acoust Soc Am 1998;103:1598–1608.

15 Yates GK, Winter IM, Robertson D: Basilar membrane nonlinearity determines auditory nerve rate-intensity functions and cochlear dynamic range. Hear Res 1990;45:203–220.

16 Ruggero MA, Robles L, Rich NC: Two-tone suppression in the basilar membrane of the cochlea: Mechanical basis of auditory-nerve rate suppression. J Neurophysiol 1992;68:1087–1099.

ORL

ORL 1999;61:305–310

3D-Finite Element Model of the Human Cochlea Including Fluid-Structure Couplings

Frank Böhnke Wolfgang Arnold

Department of Otolaryngology, Technical University of Munich, Germany

Key Words
Cochlea · Perilymph · Basilar membrane · Finite element method · Wave propagation

Abstract
The propagation of acoustic waves in the inner ear in vivo could not be quantified completely yet. This is in particular true in conjunction with the micromechanical structures of the organ of Corti, though these data are important for the explanation and discussion of clinical measurements like otoacoustic emissions and auditory brainstem responses. To access these problems a three-dimensional mechanical model of the cochlea including the fluid-structure couplings is developed and evaluated numerically by finite elements. Although the complex cochlear partition is covered by passive mechanical elements, the results fit early experiments (1928), which studied the wave propagation in the cochlea with fresh human cadavers [G. von Békésy: Experiments in Hearing. New York, McGraw-Hill, 1960]. Additionally it is now easy to calculate the mechanical input impedance of the cochlea. These results agree with recent experiments [S.N. Merchant et al.: Hear Res 1996;97:30–45].

Introduction

The human ear processes acoustic signals for communication, warning and pleasure. It consists mainly of the outer ear canal, the middle and the inner ear and the central auditory system. The inner ear is separated into the vestibular system, which is necessary for orientation in space, and the cochlea (Latin: *cochlea*, the snail), which is able to detect pressure with a frequency bandwidth of 10 octaves (20 Hz–20 kHz) and a dynamic range of 120 dB ($F = 10^6$) in its healthy state.

The human cochlea has a spiral form with 2.5 windings. Its largest dimension is only about 4 mm and its straight average length is 34 mm. The cochlea consists of three channels which are filled with lymph. Two of these channels are separated by the cochlear partition which consists of the basilar membrane, the organ of Corti, the stereocilia and the tectorial membrane. The organ of Corti contains about 3,000 inner hair cells, which transform mechanical displacements into electrical currents, about 12,000 outer hair cells and a large number of mainly supporting cells. All these cells work together highly nonlinear. However, their precise interaction is not completely understood.

For understanding the complex processes in the cochlea, the development and evaluation of a structural mechanical finite element model is presented. The peri-

KARGER

Fax + 41 61 306 12 34
E-Mail karger@karger.ch
www.karger.com

© 1999 S. Karger AG, Basel
0301–1569/99/0615–0305$17.50/0

Accessible online at:
http://BioMedNet.com/karger

Dr.-Ing. Frank Böhnke
Department of Otolaryngology
Technical University of Munich
Ismaningerstrasse 22
D–81675 München (Germany)

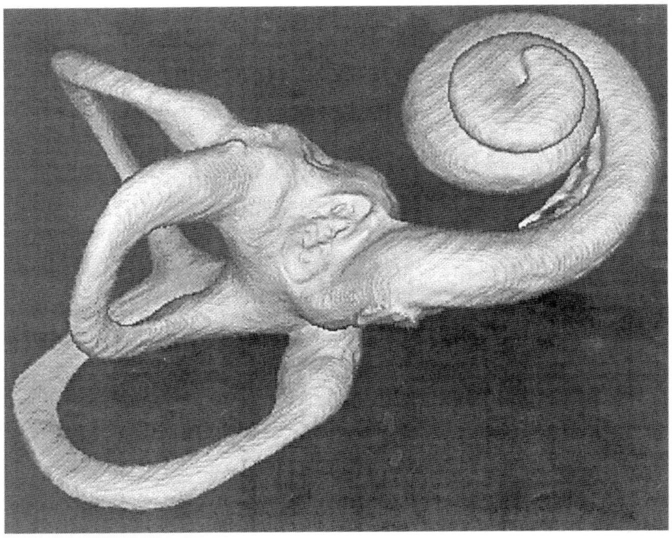

Fig. 1. Mictrotomographic image of the fluid-filled caves of the human inner ear.

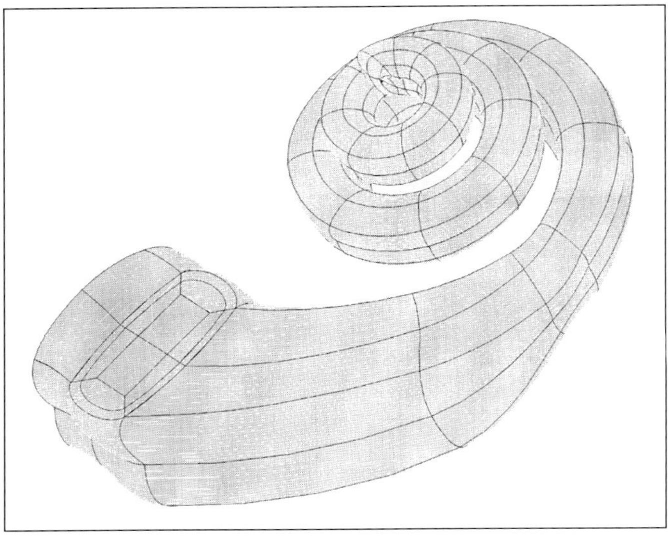

Fig. 2. Geometric model of the scala tympani and scala vestibuli of the human cochlea.

lymph is considered as inviscous and compressible. The fluid-structure couplings between the perilymph and the stapes footplate, the round window membrane and the elastic cochlear partition are covered in three dimensions for the first time.

Morphology and Methods

Figure 1 is a microtomographic image of the fluid-filled caves of the human inner ear. Further information on the imaging of microtomographic pictures are given in this issue [1].

To simulate the propagation of mechanical waves in the human cochlea we developed a three-dimensional finite element model which neglects micromechanical elements of the cochlear partition for the moment, but takes the three-dimensional fluid-structure system with its curved geometry into consideration [2]. The three-dimensional mechanical model of the cochlea is shown in figure 2. The areas which cover the kidney-shaped cross-sections of the scala vestibuli and scala tympani are located to form the curved geometry of the cochlea. The points on the boundary of these cross-sections are connected by spline functions. Because the model is built by a low number of volumes (240), inadmissibly high curvatures may result. Therefore the maximum physically permissible warping factors, which are given by the finite element package, must not be exceeded.

Cochlear Partition

The cochlear partition is idealized by two orthotropic elastic shells with variable width (80–500 μm) and thickness (7.5–2.5 μm) from the base (stapes) to the apex (helicotrema) of the cochlea [3]. The cochlear partition is divided into two identical shells because the fluid can be coupled to the upper or lower area of the shell solely with the used FE package. Their Young's moduli are E_x = 100 MPa in the transverse and E_y = 10 kPa in the longitudinal direction according to the stiff fibers embedded into the softer tissue of the basilar membrane. Of course, the areas of the shells which are on the opposite side of the adjoining fluid are coupled among themselves. Figure 3 shows one of these shells which represents the cochlear partition. The continuous decrease of thickness and the increasing width from base to apex can be seen.

All Poisson's ratios (tranverse expansions) of the shell are set to zero for the moment. This may result in a reduced accuracy of the shell dynamics when the displacement based finite elements are used because the elements may lock [4]. The damping is included specifically as material damping of the shell and chosen as $\beta = 10^{-5}$. It is worth noting that this is the only damping considered and therefore the cause for complex displacements and the phase shifts, which are found in the results.

Stapes Footplate of the Oval Window and the Round Window Membrane

The Young's modulus of the shell which represents the stapes footplate is E_{St} = 12 GPa. The Young's modulus of the annular ligament is E_{AL} = 700 kPa, which was determined experimentally for elastin [5]. The round window membrane is idealized by an elastic shell with the lower Young's modulus E_{RW} = 9.8 MPa and an average thickness t_{RW} = 100 μm. The lowest thickness was determined to 56 μm in the center of the round window membrane [6].

Perilymphatic Fluid

For simplification, only two (scala tympani, scala vestibuli) of the three fluid-filled channels (scala tympani, scala vestibuli and scala media) are taken into account. The fluid is considered as linear,

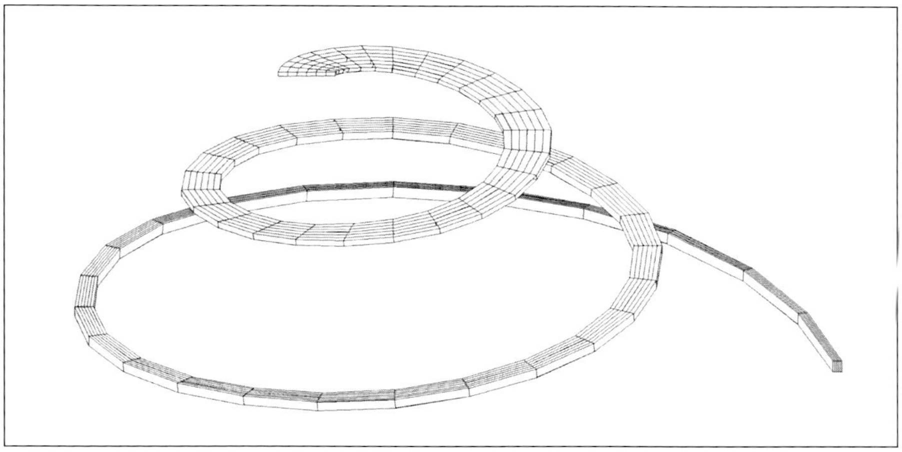

Fig. 3. Curved orthotropic shell representing the basilar membrane. The thickness at the base is 7.5 μm and continuously decreasing to 2.5 μm at the helicotrema, which are half the values of the human basilar membrane. The width is continuously increasing from 80 μm at the base of the cochlea to 500 μm near the helicotrema.

inviscous and compressible and therefore we are able to cover fast acoustic waves in the fluid. The bulk modulus K of the perilymphatic fluid is equal to that of water K = 2,250 MPa. With the fluid density $\rho_{Fl} = 10^3$ *[kg/m³]* the speed of sound in the fluid is:

$$c_{Fl} = \sqrt{\frac{K}{\rho_{Fl}}} = 1{,}500\,\frac{m}{s} \qquad (1)$$

Fluid-Structure Coupling

It is necessary to couple the areas of the stapes footplate, the area of the round window and both areas of the cochlear partition (upper and lower) to the lymph. Because the location of the oval and the round window are not orthogonal to the global Cartesian coordinate system, two additional local Cartesian coordinate systems must be introduced. Because shell elements may be coupled to the fluid with only one of their areas, the cochlear partition is represented by two double-curved shells. In each case the outer shell areas are coupled to the fluid. On the opposite sides the shells are coupled to each other and their distance is adjustable.

Figure 4 shows the complete cochlear model discretized with finite elements. The chosen discretization leads to approximately 32,000 finite elements and therefore about 115,000 variables (active degrees of freedom) must be evaluated.

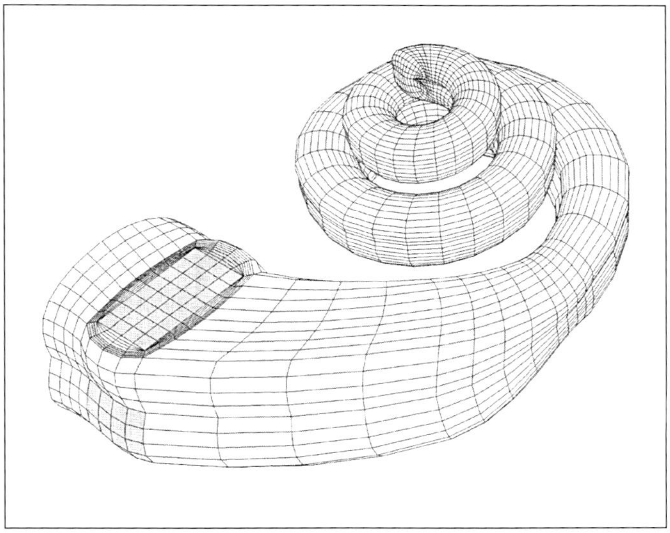

Fig. 4. Cochlear model discretized with finite elements.

Boundary Conditions

To solve the problem numerically, appropriate boundary conditions must be introduced. The perilymph is enclosed by rigid bone. Therefore, the normal components of the fluid displacements must vanish at the bony surrounding areas. Because the fluid is assumed to be inviscous the tangential components do not vanish. If viscosity is covered it is essential to use special boundary conditions, which cover the vanishing of all displacement components at rigid walls.

The shells which represent the cochlear partition must be supported correctly. The inner boundary at the lamina spiralis ossea is clamped and therefore all displacements and rotations vanish there. On the opposite side at the ligamentum spirale, the shells are simply supported. Therefore, rotations relating to the longitudinal (cochlea) direction may be different from zero. Rotations relating to the two axes orthogonal to the longitudinal axis and all displacements vanish at the outer border of the shells at the ligamentum spirale.

The boundaries of the shell, which represents the round window, are clamped. Therefore, all displacements and rotations vanish at the rim of the round window.

Acoustic Input Impedance of the Cochlea

The acoustic input impedance Z_C of the cochlea is defined as the ratio between the pressure P_S at the stapes footplate and the velocity v_S of the displaced volume. Under the assumption of harmonic excitation, this ratio becomes:

$$Z_C = \frac{P_S}{j\omega X_S A_S} \qquad (2)$$

X_S is the displacement of the stapes in z-direction, A_S is the stapes area, ω is the circular frequency and j is the imaginary unit indicating a complex value.

Results

Wave Propagation in the Cochlea

The external load is applied as a pressure on the stapes footplate area. Its amplitude is $P_S = 1$ Pa, which is equal to the sound pressure level $L_e = 94$ dB(SPL) in all cases.

Our results show calculations using external harmonic loads of three different frequencies: $f_1 = 100$ Hz, $f_2 = 2{,}000$ Hz and $f_3 = 10{,}000$ Hz. The frequency range is not limited, and therefore a static analysis and a frequency, e.g. f = 20,000 Hz, could additionally be applied.

For the external pressure with the lowest frequency $f_1 = 100$ Hz, the maximum absolute value of the displacement (0.14 nm) of the cochlear partition is at a distance of 30 mm from the stapes footplate near the helicotrema (fig. 5a). The horizontal line marks the constant phase shift. The whole cochlear partition is moving in phase. The phase is independent of the locus along the cochlear partition. Figure 5b shows the pressure distribution at the cochlear partition for the same frequency. The absolute value of the pressure decreases continuously from 0.08 Pa to a value near 0 Pa with a constant phase shift.

A harmonic pressure of frequency $f_2 = 2{,}000$ Hz at the stapes footplate leads to a maximum displacement (0.2 nm) of the cochlear partition at approximately half the cochlea length (fig. 6a). In this case the maximum phase shift is at least –2,160° or $-12\,\pi$. The pressure is mainly decreasing from the stapes (0.016 Pa) to the helicotrema to a pressure near 0 Pa (fig. 6b, upper line). It is interesting to note that the phase of the pressure (fig. 6b, lower line) has both negative and positive slopes and does not exceed $-1.5\,\pi$. At $f_3 = 10$ kHz the maximum absolute value of the displacement (0.23 nm) is at a distance of only 5 mm from the stapes footplate and the maximum phase shift is about –360° or $-2\,\pi$ (fig. 7a). The pressure decreases from 0.33 Pa at the stapes to a value near 0 Pa at the helicotrema. There are only low variations of the pressure phase from the constant shift ($-0.6\,\pi$) in the basal part of the cochlea (fig. 7b, lower line).

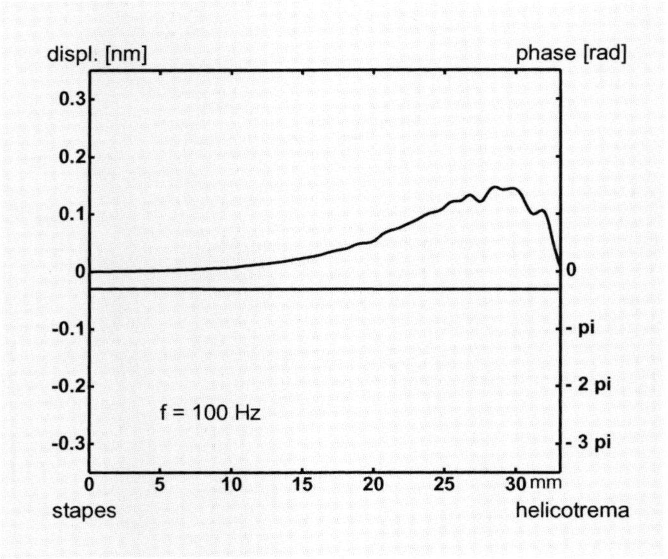

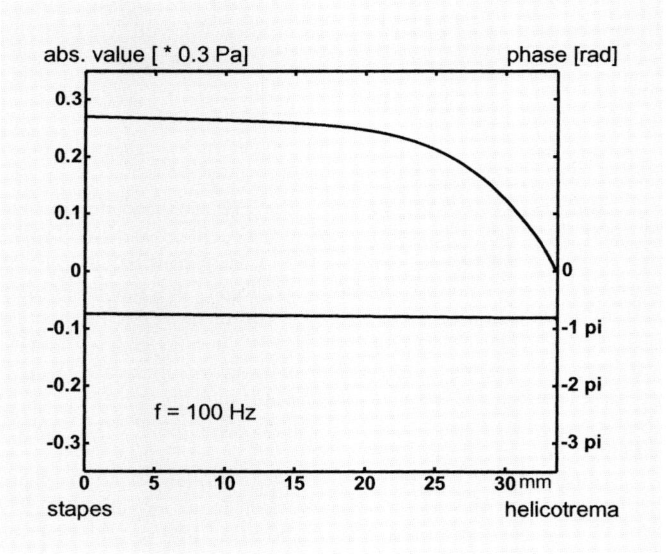

Fig. 5. a Absolute displacement and phase of displacement along the cochlear partition with external pressure amplitude 1 Pa and frequency $f_1 = 100$ Hz. **b** Absolute pressure and phase of pressure at the cochlear partition with external pressure amplitude 1 Pa and frequency $f_1 = 100$ Hz.

Acoustic Input Impedance of the Cochlea

For an external pressure of frequency f = 1,000 Hz and amplitude 1 Pa at the stapes footplate, the displacement of the stapes footplate is evaluated to 0.2 nm, which is also determined from temporal bones of human cadavers [7]. It is interesting to note that this is only twice the diameter of an atom. If the area of the stapes footplate is chosen as $A_s = 3.6$ mm^2, the acoustic input impedance of the cochlea model is:

$$Z_C = -j\,138.89 \cdot 10^9 \text{ Pa s/m}^3 = -j\,138.89 \text{ G}\Omega$$

which is the stiffness component. This value is a factor 1.38 above the experimental value [7] and therefore in close proximity. The derived unit ohm (Ω) indicates the acoustic impedance in the meter-kilogram-second (mks) system.

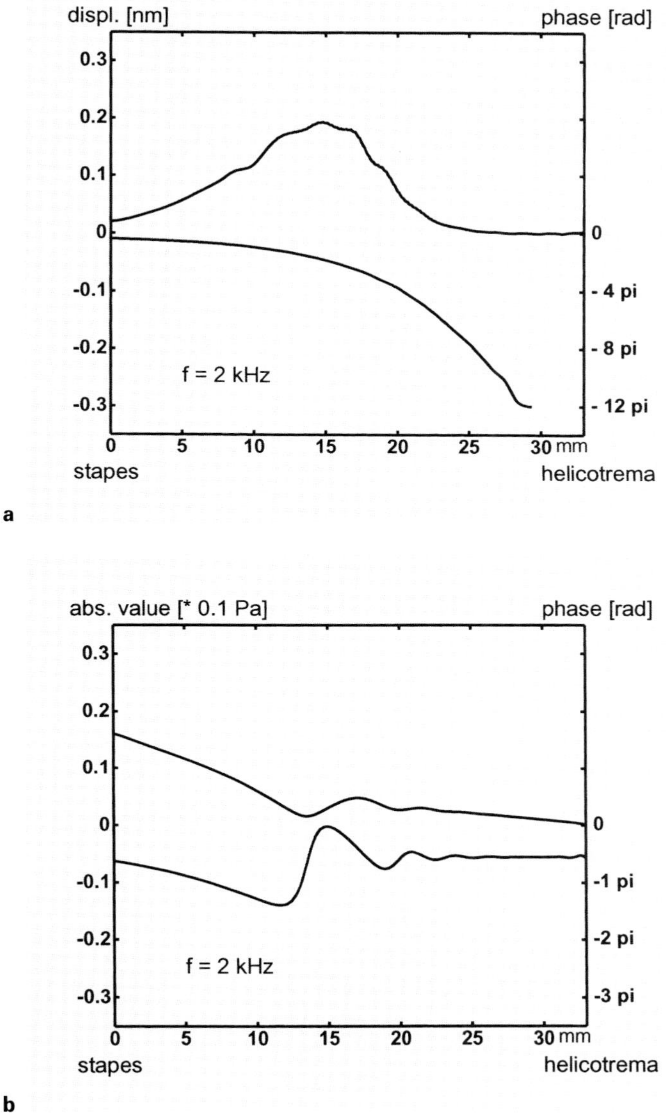

Fig. 6. a Absolute displacement and phase of displacement along the cochlear partition with external pressure amplitude 1 Pa and frequency f_2 = 2,000 Hz. **b** Absolute pressure and phase of pressure at the cochlear partition with external pressure amplitude 1 Pa and frequency f_2 = 2,000 Hz.

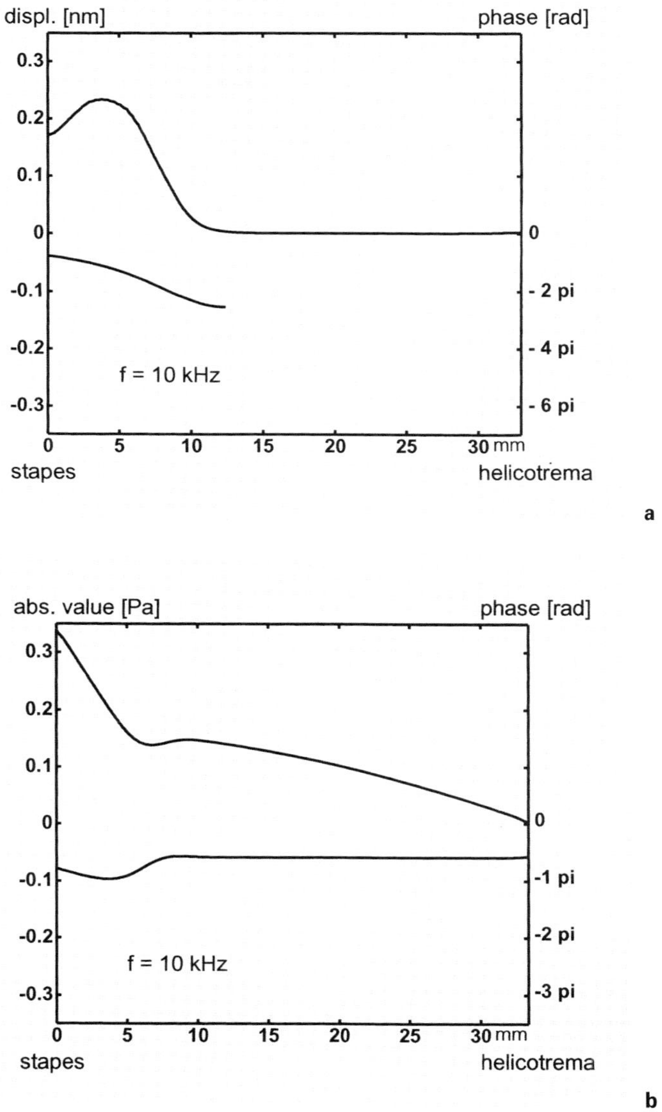

Fig. 7. a Absolute displacement and phase of displacement along the cochlear partition with external pressure amplitude 1 Pa and frequency f_3 = 10,000 Hz. **b** Absolute pressure and phase of pressure at the cochlear partition with external pressure amplitude 1 Pa and frequency f_3 = 10,000 Hz.

Discussion

The calculated displacements and pressures are those we expect in comparison with former experiments [7, 8]. The question for the existence of traveling or standing waves can now easily be answered. The damping, which is material damping here solely, is the cause for phase shifts of the displacement of the cochlear partition and the pressure in the lymph. If the damping is neglected, real displacements and pressures result and in this case we find standing waves in the cochlea.

It is interesting to note that the maximum displacement of the basilar membrane is of the same order of magnitude (0.2 nm) for the three frequencies, which span a frequency bandwidth of more than 6 octaves. This is in contrast to the values for the pressure. We assume this is a consequence of the dimensions of the basilar membrane, which increases in width and decreases in thickness from the base to the apex of the cochlea respectively.

The acoustic input impedance of the cochlea can be determined numerically now. This is relevant for the realistic termination of middle ear models. A good agreement with recent experimental values is found. The evaluated displacement of the stapes footplate is only 0.2 nm with an external applied pressure L_e = 94 dB(SPL) at the stapes footplate (f = 1,000 Hz). If an increase of the pressure caused by the middle ear by 20 dB is assumed, this displacement (0.2 nm) corresponds to 74 dB(SPL) in the ear canal. The linear extrapolation of the stapes displacement leads to an extremely small value for the hearing threshold at L_{HS} = 0 dB(SPL), namely 0.04 pm (picometer) or 40 fm (femtometer, Fermi).

In a future investigation, the acoustic input impedance of the cochlea will be evaluated in a wider frequency range (20–20,000 Hz).

Because the viscosity of the fluid cannot be included easily in a curved geometry by the finite element package used, we are unable to calculate shearing forces in the fluid. As a consequence, an incompatibility in the formulation of the fluid-structure system results because the equations describing the mechanical behavior of the shell contain rotations. These cannot be coupled to a fluid which is described by displacements and pressure solely.

Conclusions

(1) The 3D-finite element model allows the evaluation of the passive mechanical behavior of the human cochlea with arbitrary input pressure at the stapes footplate including all kinds of slow and fast waves in the lymph and the cochlear partition.

(2) The curved geometry of the cochlea and the fluid-structure coupling is covered in three dimensions. Therefore, the micromechanical structures of the organ of Corti and those of the cochlear partition can be easily included in further investigations.

(3) The linear solutions are in close agreement with early experimental results taken from human temporal bones [8]. To cover the nonlinear physical behavior of the cochlea, material and geometrical nonlinearities should be included in future calculations.

Acknowledgements

We gratefully acknowledge the support of Dr. R. Schmidt (TU-Dresden) and of CADFEM in Grafing (Germany) in helping us using the ANSYS 5.4 finite element software.

References

1 Vogel U: New approach for 3D-imaging and geometry modeling of the human inner ear. ORL 1999;61:259–267.
2 Böhnke F, Schmidt R: Aspekte der FE-Modellierung der Hörschnecke des Menschen. Proc 15th CAD-FEM Users' Meeting, Fulda, Germany, Oct. 1997, pp 1–11.
3 Wada H, Sugawara M, Kobayashi T, Hozawa K, Takasaka T: Measurement of guinea pig basilar membrane using computer-aided three-dimensional reconstruction system. Hear Res 1998;120:1–6.
4 Bathe KJ: Finite Element Procedures. Englewood Cliffs, Prentice-Hall, 1996.
5 Carton RW, Dainauskas J, Clark JW: Elastic properties of single elastic fibres. J Appl Physiol 1962;17:547–551.
6 Nomura Y: Otological Significance of the Round Window. Adv Otorhinolaryngol. Basel, Karger, 1984, vol 33, pp 1–162.
7 Merchant SN, Ravicz ME, Rosowski JJ: Acoustic input impedance of the stapes and cochlea in human temporal bones. Hear Res 1996;97:30–45.
8 von Békésy G: Experiments in Hearing. New York, McGraw-Hill, 1960.

ORL

ORL 1999;61:311–317

Active Nonlinear Mechanics of the Organ of Corti Including the Stereocilia-Tectorial Membrane Complex

Frank Böhnke Jutta von Mikusch-Buchberg Wolfgang Arnold

Department of Otolaryngology, Technical University of Munich, Germany

Key Words
Organ of Corti · Cochlear amplifier · Outer hair cell · Nonlinearity · Stereocilia · Tectorial membrane

Abstract
There is a large amount of knowledge about the different components of the organ of Corti (OC), but little is known about how these components act together in vivo. To clarify the complex mechanical behavior of the OC, anatomic results are carefully analyzed and used to develop a finite element model of a short section of OC, which includes 8 outer hair cells (OHC) and their supporting structures. The modal analysis shows the frequency-dependent phase reversal of the radial stereocilia displacement. The transient computation confirms the amplification of OC displacements when the ability of the OHC to contract and elongate is considered. The inclusion of a nonlinear function describing the mechanoelectrical transduction in OHC amplifies and distorts the displacement of the OC when it is stimulated by a sinusoidal input pressure function. These results are in agreement with other psychoacoustic, electrophysiologic and otoacoustic measurements.

Introduction

Though intense research has been conducted on the micromechanics of the organ of Corti (OC) since its discovery [1], the in vivo behavior remains unclear. One of the reasons for this is that it is difficult to yield mechanical parameters, e.g. Young's modulus, of the heterogeneous cell composition, using in vivo measurements. In addition to that, modern computers are not able to calculate the biomechanics of the cochlea including the complete OC with its million degrees of freedom. Therefore, former simulations of cochlear mechanics either neglected known anatomical details or considered only a small number of cells from the complete system. To clarify the complex signal transduction process in the cochlea, we developed a three-dimensional finite element (3D-FE) model of the OC including the stereocilia (St) and the tectorial membrane (TM). While the study neglects wave propagation effects, it resolves details of the cochlear partition, which divides the fluid-filled channels scala media and scala tympani. The stereocilia displacement and the resulting mechanoelectric transduction is caused by the shearing of the TM relative to the reticular lamina (RL) in the transverse direction, i.e. perpendicular to the main direction of wave propagation in the longitudinal direction of the cochlea.

The reader is referred to other contemporary literature concerning cochlear modelling [2, 3].

KARGER

Fax + 41 61 306 12 34
E-Mail karger@karger.ch
www.karger.com

© 1999 S. Karger AG, Basel
0301–1569/99/0615–0311$17.50/0

Accessible online at:
http://BioMedNet.com/karger

Dr.-Ing. Frank Böhnke
Department of Otolaryngology
Technical University of Munich
Ismaningerstrasse 22
D–81675 München (Germany)

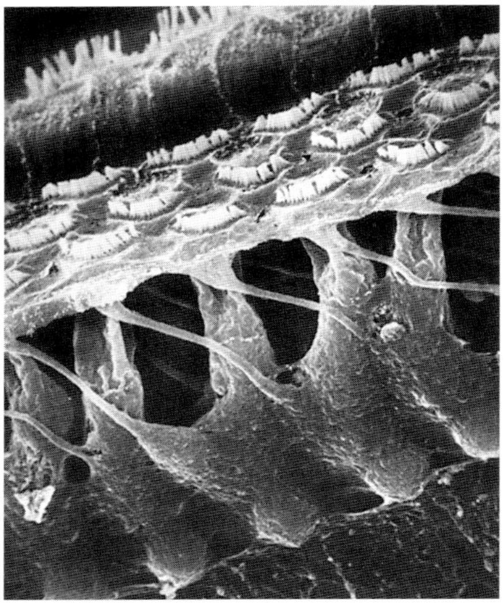

Fig. 1. SEM of OHC supported by Php of DC.

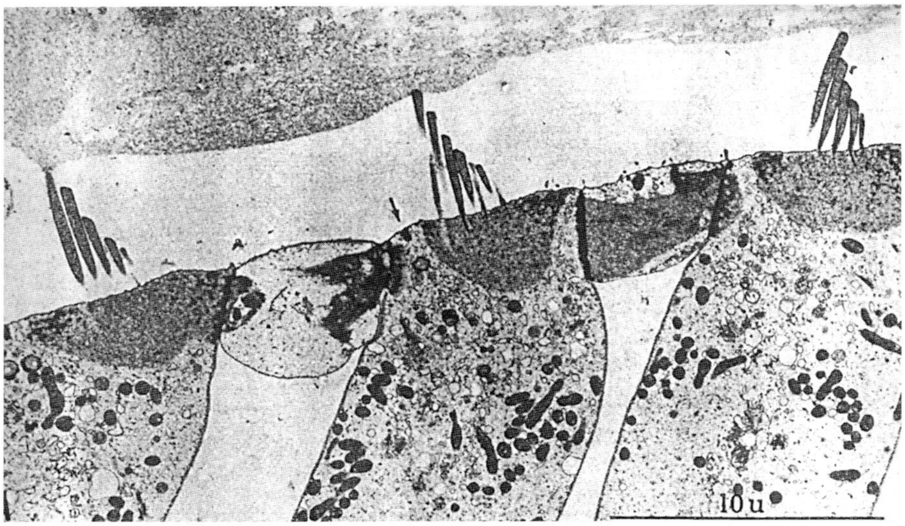

Fig. 2. Coupling of the longest St of OHC to the TM.

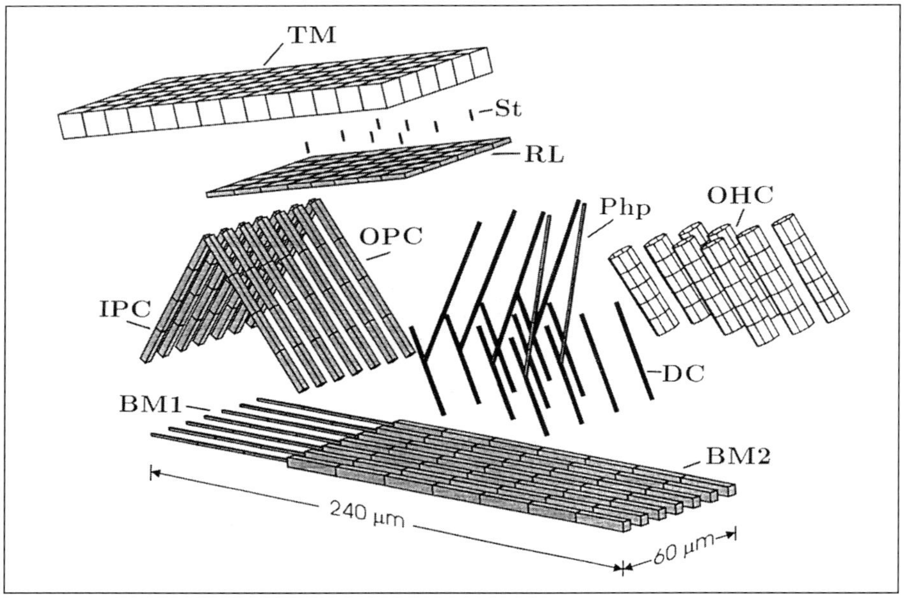

Fig. 3. Components of the FE model with 8 OHC.

Morphology and Methods

A small section of the OC that includes only 8 of the approximately 12,000 outer hair cells (OHCs) of a human cochlea is considered. The surrounding lymphatic fluid is not included in the model, but its mechanical effect is approximated by the symmetrical loading of the organ. Anatomical results used during the development of the FE model have been described previously [4]. Figure 1 shows a scanning electron microscopic (SEM) image of the OC, including the staggered positions of the OHCs. On top of each OHC, the w-shaped form of the stereocilia bundles can be seen. The phalangeal processes (Php) of Deiters' cells (DC) are clearly visible. One Php runs from the head of an OHC to the base of the next but one OHC. The Php are slender bodies (length ≈ 70 μm >> diameter ≈ 1 μm) of fibers that are constructed with the protein f-actin. The junctions between the stereocilia of three OHC and the TM are shown at a high magnification in figure 2 [5]. Only the longest stereocilia of the bundles, i.e. those corresponding to the outermost row of bundles, are connected to the TM. Figure 3 shows the different components of the resulting FE model of the small section ($l = 60$ μm) of the OC.

The basilar membrane (BM) constitutes the base of the system on which the OC is located. To circumvent difficulties with the idealization of the BM as an orthotropic shell, e.g. the unknown shearing modulus and Poisson ratios of the shell, it is represented by a set of 14 beams (7 pairs). Each transversal fiber is represented using two rectangular beams of different widths [1 μm (BM1) and 4 μm (BM2)] to reflect accurately anatomical results. The complete length of one beam pair is l_{BM} = 240 μm representing a medial part of the human BM. Young's modulus of these beams is chosen as 1.7 GPa according to static point load measurements in the basal part of the guinea pig cochlea [6].

The inner (IPC) and outer pillar cells (OPC) are idealized as straight elastic beams (length = 71.8 μm, width = 3 μm).

The DC support the OHC and are represented as thin (1 μm) beams. They consist of Deiters' rods (l_{rod} = 38.5 μm) and their Php (l_{Php} = 62.9 μm). Their average Young's modulus was recently determined again (E_{DC} = 45 MPa) [7].

The OHC are idealized as straight isotropic elastic pipes with wall thicknesses of 0.1 μm and E_{OHC} = 45 kPa [8]. The average length is 55 μm. Their natural ability to elongate and contract is modelled by heating and cooling according to a thermal expansion coefficient $\alpha = 10^{-4}$. This feature can be switched on or off to simulate the active or passive OC, respectively. To yield an effective gain of 40 dB for the displacement of the RL, an OHC gain of $g \approx 2$ (i.e. the ratio of somatic OHC length change to stereocilia bundle displacement; fig. 4) is chosen. This reflects other experimental results [9].

The RL consists of the endings of the OHC and the Php and the junction between the upper parts of the IPC and OPC. It is idealized as an isotropic plate ($A = 60 \times 104$ μm, E_{RL} = 1.7 GPa). The head of the IPC and OPC is firmly attached.

The TM is idealized as a structural solid and discretized with 3D 8-node finite elements with three displacements and three rotations per node. Its Young's modulus is chosen as E_{TM} = 30 kPa which is the value given for the TM of the bobtail lizard [10]. The density is ρ_{TM} = 1 mg/mm^3 as it is in all other cases. Therefore, the mass of the TM is included.

The St are covered as elastic beams whose Young's modulus is 20 MPa and their lengths and diameters are 4 and 0.2 μm, respectively.

The complete system of equations used to calculate the 3D-FE model contains 2,298 variables, which are displacements and rotations. For the transient computation (see Results) a symmetric external load is used. It consists of a pressure acting on top of the TM surface and 11 forces acting on the nodes of the BM beams.

Nonlinear OHC Function

The nonlinear processing of acoustic signals by the ear has been verified by psychoacoustical observations, electrophysiological examinations and the analysis of the saturating behavior of evoked otoacoustic emissions, but the sources of the nonlinearities remained unidentified. Possible sources include: material, geometrical (the dependence of the stiffness on the displacement) and state-dependent nonlinearities of mechanical structures, the nonlinear mechanoelectrical transduction process of auditory hair cells and nonlinear neural coding of information, e.g. rate intensity functions. A mixture of all these nonlinearities is effective in vivo and it is difficult to distinguish separate causes. Because geometrical nonlinearities are expected to be relevant at high levels (>80 dB SPL) and material nonlinearities are not yet quantified, the nonlinear OHC function is solely used in the present study.

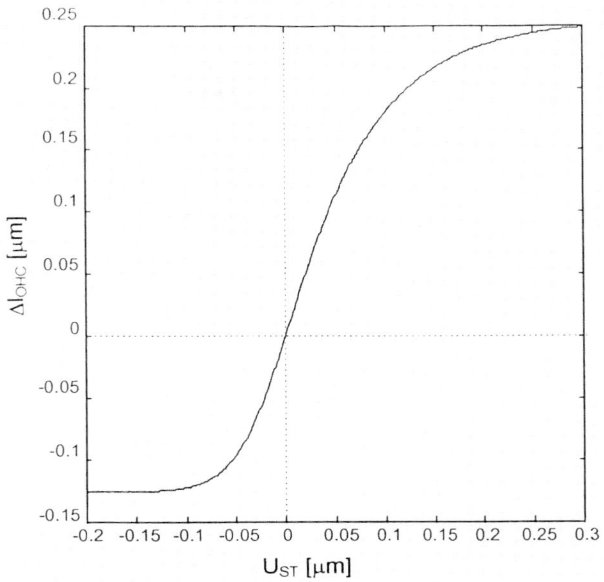

Fig. 4. Asymmetric nonlinear transfer function of the OHC length to the St displacement.

The alternating component of the receptor potential ΔV_r as a function of the stereocilia displacement u_{St} is given by a second-order Boltzmann function, which was developed based on statistical considerations [11]:

$$\Delta V_r = \frac{V_{SS}}{1 + e^{-C_1(u_{St} - u_1)/kT}\left(1 + e^{-C_2(u_{St} - u_2)/kT}\right)} - V_H \qquad (1)$$

V_{SS} is the peak-to-peak value and V_H is the membrane potential for maximal hyperpolarization. The constants C_1 and C_2 were determined as $C_1 = 60\ fN$ and $C_2 = 120\ fN$ and u_1 = 56.8 nm and u_2 = 27.3 nm, respectively [12]. The product kT can be calculated with the Boltzmann constant k and the temperature T. Taking the multiple elementary motor model of the OHC wall into consideration [13], an axial length change as a function of the alternating receptor potential ΔV_r is given by:

$$\Delta l_{OHC} = c_0 L_0 N \left(\frac{1}{1 + e^{-\Delta V_r a_0 + b_0}} - \frac{1}{1 + e^{b_0}}\right) \qquad (2)$$

with L_0 = 55 μm the OHC (quiet)-length, N = 80 μm^{-1} the packing density of elementary motors and three constants a_0 = 0.009 mV^{-1}, b_0 = 1.45 and c_0 = 0.18 nm. Figure 4 shows the asymmetrical transfer function of the OHC length change Δl_{OHC} as a function of the stereocilia displacement, which may be approximated by a linear function of slope $s = 2$, equivalent to the gain, g, in its origin.

According to the low frequency cut-off of the receptor potential of the mammalian OHC, filters with different low frequency cut-offs were included in the feedback path of the active system. Though the stability of the system depends on this parameter, the results shown in figures 7–9 are calculated without the use of frequency-limiting filters.

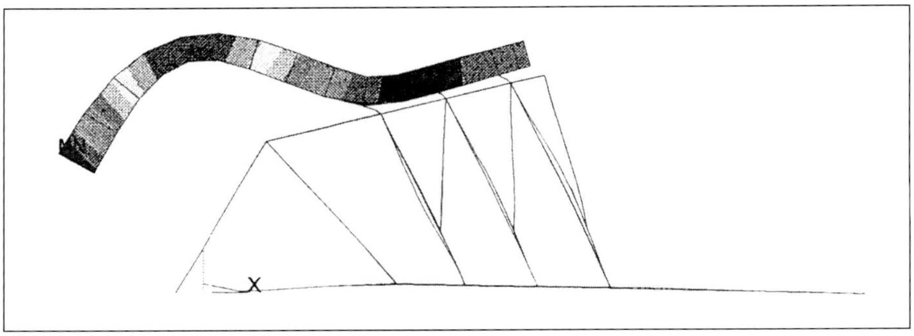

Fig. 5. Displaced structure (first eigenfrequency f_1 = 3,585.7 Hz).

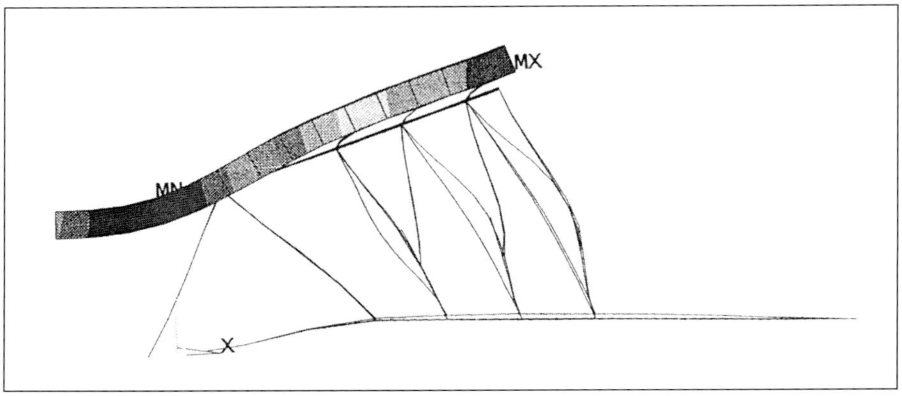

Fig. 6. Displaced structure (second eigenfrequency f_2 = 6,841.8 Hz).

Results

Modal Analysis

In order to calculate eigenfrequencies and eigenvalues of the system with 8 OHCs, a damped modal analysis is used. The damping is included by material damping for all elements (damping factor $\beta = 10^{-5}$). Figure 5 shows the displaced system (eigenvalues) for the first eigenfrequency (f_1 = 3,585.7 Hz). The displacement of the BM towards scala vestibuli (up) results in the stereocilia heads being deflected to the left (negative x-direction), whereas the direction of the stereocilia heads deflection is reversed when the eigenvalues of the second mode (f_2 = 6,841.8 Hz) are used (fig. 6). This result is in agreement with the former proposal of Zwislocki [14], who suggested a phase reversal by interpreting neurophysiological data. As shown in figure 6, the displacement of the TM in z-direction is maximal at the place of the stereocilia of the inner hair cell. This result may differ if additional coupling structures are included here. Hints for this anatomical detail concerning the coupling of the stereocilia of inner hair cells to Hensen's stripe of the TM were given by Lim [15], but the real in vivo conditions remain controversial, at least for the human cochlea.

Transient Computation

In figures 7–9, respectively, the displacements of the RL (z-direction, near the outermost OHC, gray), the displacements of the BM (z-direction, center of the BM plane, black), and the horizontal deflection of the stereocilia head of an OHC (x-direction, light gray) are shown in case of a switched sinusoidal excitation (L = 40 dB SPL). In the passive case, using the frequency f_{ext} = 1,000 Hz (fig. 7), the deflection of the BM towards scala vestibuli (up) results in a deflection of the stereocilia head to the right (positive x-direction); this corresponds with the classical shearing between TM and RL originally proposed by ter Kuile [16] and given later in a clear representation [17]. In this passive case, with the frequency of excitation below the first eigenfrequency, the amplitude of the RL displacement is 0.22 nm.

When the organ is excited with an external signal of the first eigenfrequency (f_1 = 3,585.7 Hz), the amplitude of the RL displacement increases to 1.5 nm due to resonance and the displacement of the stereocilia head changes its sign relative to the BM displacement in the z-direction (fig. 8). When the activity of the OHC is considered, a further increase of the RL displacement (40 dB, amplitude = 160 nm) results (fig. 9), and a considerable amount of dis-

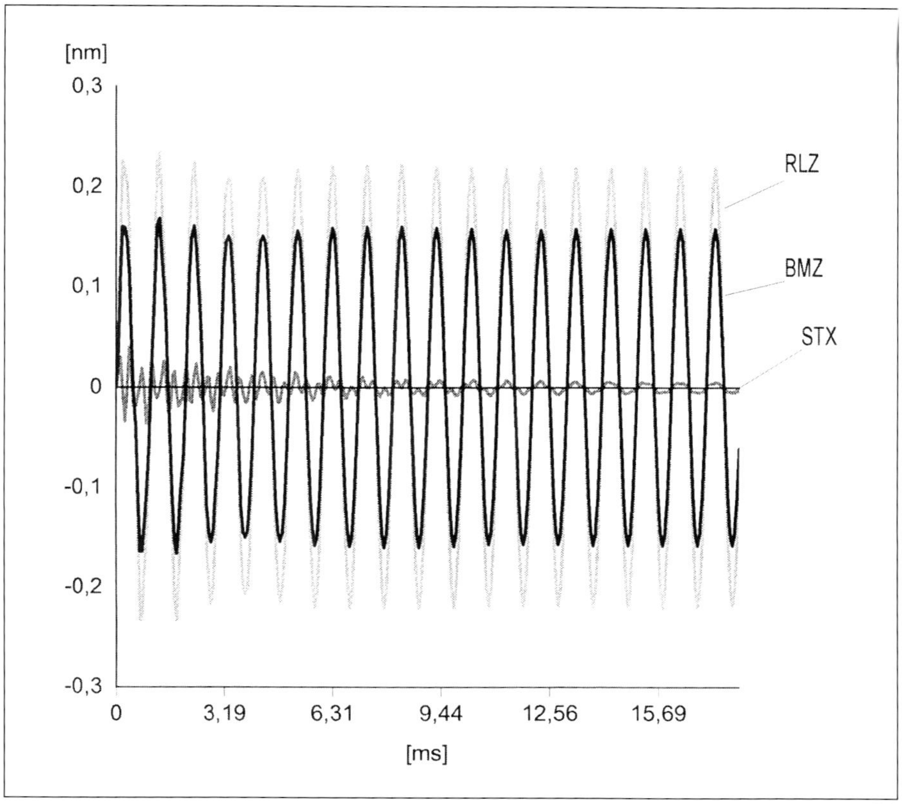

Fig. 7. z-Displacement of the BM (BMZ), RL (RLZ) and x-displacement of St (STX) for f_{ext} = 1,000 Hz of the passive OC.

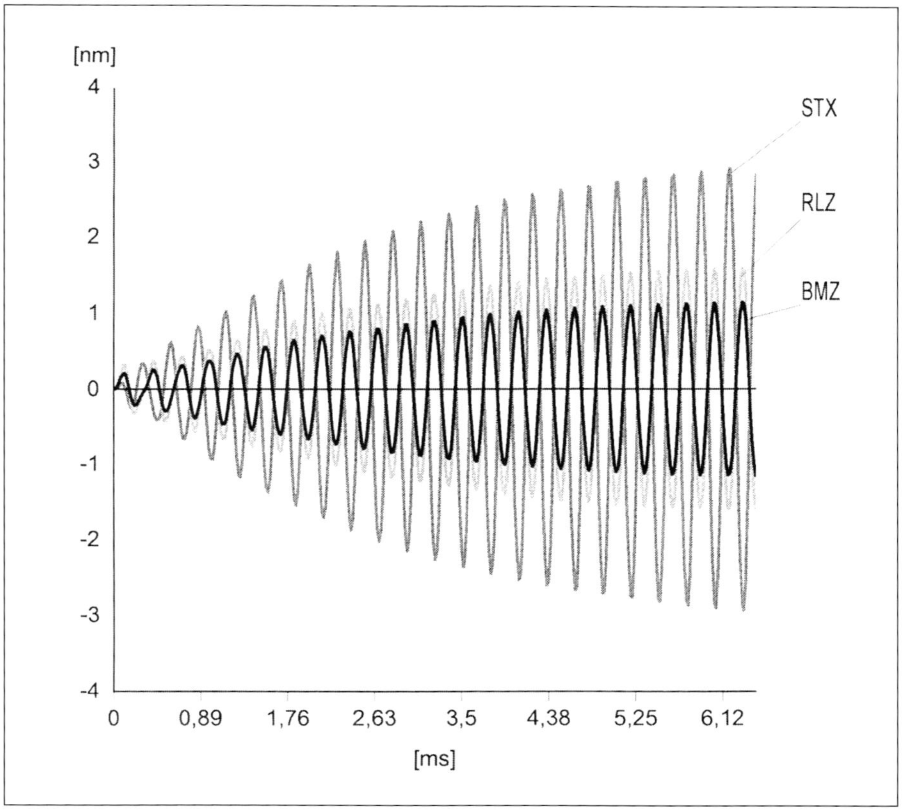

Fig. 8. z-Displacement of the BM (BMZ), RL (RLZ) and x-displacement of St (STX) for f_{ext} = 3,585.7 Hz of the passive OC.

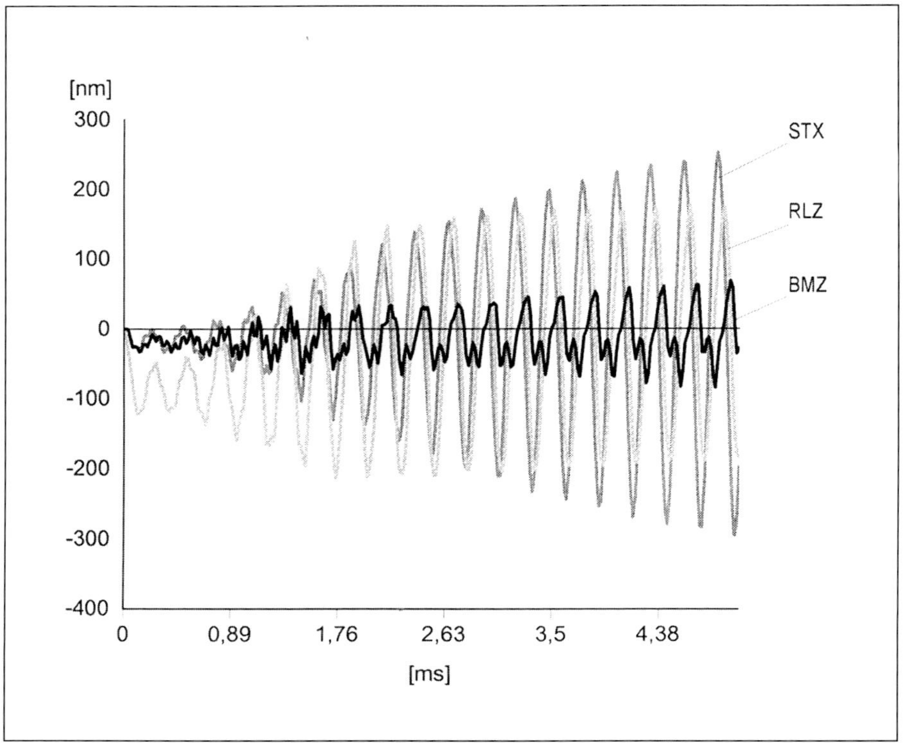

Fig. 9. z-Displacement of the BM (BMZ), RL (RLZ) and x-displacement of St (STX) for f_{ext} = 3,585.7 Hz of the active OC.

tortion, especially of the BM motion, can be seen. Thus, the displacement of the OC is amplified and distorted by the active processing of the OHC.

Discussion

The results of this study support the hypothesis of the cochlear amplifier [18, 19]. The inclusion of the OHC as active mechatronical elements in a FE model produces a 40 dB amplification of the displacement of the OC. This amplification is achieved though the OHC gain (or mechanomotility) is only $g \approx 2$. In order to explain this, it may be useful to consider the involved energies. While only a small amount of energy is necessary to displace the heads of the stereocila bundle, considerably more energy is needed to displace the whole OC. Because the cochlear partition realizes a positive feedback system for specific places and frequencies, an amplification of energy occurs. As a result, the activity enables the OC to overcome internal friction and viscous forces; this is a necessity for hearing at very low sound pressure levels. The energy is provided by the biological battery located in the stria vascularis.

The amplification is reduced by the destruction or pathologies of the OHC. This is in agreement with cochlear hearing losses when the OHC are damaged and fail to amplify. The psychoacoustic consequences are threshold increase and loudness recruitment. Though the nonlinear OHC transduction process is considered in this study, the resulting nonlinearity could only be presented very roughly in form of the distorted time signal (fig. 9). To further our understanding of how the OC components function, spectral analyses, variations of the external levels and nonlinear oscillations need to be studied.

References

1 Corti A: Recherches sur l'organe de l'ouïe des mammifères. Z wiss Zool 1851;3:109–169.
2 Gummer AW, Hemmert W, Zenner HP: Resonant tectorial membrane motion in the inner ear: Its crucial role in frequency tuning. Proc Natl Acad Sci USA 1996;93:8727–8732.
3 Steele Ch, Lim KM: Cochlear model with three-dimensional fluid, inner sulcus and feedforward mechanism. Audiol Neurootol 1999;4: 197–203.
4 Böhnke F, Arnold W: Studie der Auslenkungen und Rotationen des Corti-Organs in drei Dimensionen. Otorhinolaryngol Nova 1996;6: 69–77.
5 Kimura RS: Hairs of the cochlear sensory cells and their attachment to the tectorial membrane. Arch Otolaryngol 1966;61:55–72.
6 Miller CE: Structural implications of basilar membrane compliance measurements. J Acoust Soc Am 1985;77:1465–1474.
7 Laffon E, Angelini E: On the Deiters' cell contribution to the micromechanics of the organ of Corti. Hear Res 1996;99:106–109.
8 Ratnanather JT, Brownell WE, Popel AS: Mechanical Properties of the Outer Hair Cell. Biophysics of Hair Cell Sensory System. Groningen, Academisch Ziekenhuis, 1993, pp 149–155.
9 Evans BN, Dallos P: Stereocilia displacement induced somatic motility of cochlear outer hair cells. Proc Natl Acad Sci USA 1993;90:8347–8351.
10 Steele Ch: Three-Dimensional Mechanical Modeling of the Cochlea. Conference on Diversity in Auditory Mechanics, Berkeley, Calif 1996, pp 509–515.
11 Kros CJ, Rüsch A, Richardson GP: Mechanoelectrical transducer currents in hair cells of the cultured neonatal mouse cochlea. Proc R Soc Lond B 1992;249:185–193.
12 Preyer S, Gummer AW: Nonlinearity of mechanoelectrical transduction of outer hair cells as the source of nonlinear basilar-membrane motion and loudness recruitment. Audiol Neurootol 1996;1:3–11.
13 Dallos P, Hallworth R, Evans BN: Theory of electrically driven shape changes of cochlear outer hair cells. J Neurophysiol 1993;70:299–323.
14 Zwislocki JJ: Five decades of research on cochlear mechanics. J Acoust Soc Am 1980;67: 1679–1685.
15 Lim DJ: Functional structure of the organ of Corti: A review. Hear Res 1986;22:117–146.
16 ter Kuile E: Die Übertragung der Energie von der Grundmembran auf die Haarzellen. Pflügers Arch Ges Physiol 1900;79:146–157/Die richtige Bewegungsform der Membrana basilaris. Pflügers Arch Ges Physiol 1900;79:484–509.
17 Davis H: A model for transduction action in the cochlea. Cold Spring Harb Symp Quant Biol 1965;30:181–190.
18 Gold T: Hearing. II. The physical basis of the action of the cochlea. Proc Roy Soc B 1948; 135:492–498.
19 Davis H: An active process in cochlear mechanics. Hear Res 1983;9:1–49.

Author Index Vol. 61, No. 5, 1999

Subject Index Vol. 61, No. 5, 1999

KARGER

Fax +41 61 306 12 34
E-Mail karger@karger.ch
www.karger.com

© 1999 S. Karger AG, Basel

Accessible online at:
http://BioMedNet.com/karger

ORL

Joel D. Swartz, H. Ric Harnsberger

Imaging of the Temporal Bone; 3rd ed.

Thieme, Stuttgart 1998
512 pp., DM 248.–
ISBN 3-13-688403-5

The book under consideration shows a high quality in get-up, the binding is solid. We find a very large amount of modern, well-reproduced and inscribed CT and MRI scans. References are extensive; a reference list exists for every single chapter. *Imaging of the Temporal Bone* begins with an introduction in which several algorithms for the most important clinical problems are presented with the intention to standardize diagnostic procedures. The further arragement follows a topographic or clinical-anatomic scheme. External auditory canal, middle ear and inner ear structures are discussed in separate chapters. Another special chapter deals with the vessels of the temporal bone and here especially with the problem of pulsatile tinnitus, with the seventh and eighth cranial nerves and with temporal bone trauma.

Before the clinical considerations in every chapter, a detailed anatomic description is made, including schematic drawings, CT and MRI scans. In addition there are statements on embryology which are important for the understanding of pathogenetic processes. In the chapter on the external auditory canal, tumorous and inflammatory diseases are the mean topic. The following part concerning the middle ear and mastoid begins with very detailed high-resolution CT scans of the middle ear space and ossicular chain.

CT and MRI diagnosis of cholesteatoma and postoperative middle ear are the main topics in the clinical part. A special section follows showing vascular anomalies and vascular lesions of the temporal bone including an extensive discussion of pulsatile tinnitus. The opportunities of modern vessel diagnostics by means of MRI are emphasized, MR angiography and conventional angiography (digital subtraction angiography) are compared. Especially this chapter and the one concerning the facial nerve consider neurologic disorders toc. The main topics in inner ear diseases are first congenital disorders and malformations; further, otosclerosis is discussed in detail. Numerous high-resolution CTs in axial and coronal planes show different forms and phases of otosclerosis.

Considering traumatology, the consequences of longitudinal and transverse fractures of the temporal bone are shown, schematic drawings of the middle and inner ear give a clear anatomic description; traumatic lesions of the ossicular chain are emphasized. In the last part of this book, we find a special chapter concerning the disorders of the facial and vestibulocochlear nerves.

Facial nerve anatomy is described precisely from brainstem nuclei to the exit out of the stylomastoid foramen. This description might have been somewhat clearer by a continuous presentation of axial or coronal CT scans combined with schematic anatomic drawings as in other parts of this book. A lot of examples prove the growing importance of high-resolution MR techniques in temporal bone diagnostic, especially high-resolution T_2-weighted FSE sequences. Most important topics are neoplastic diseases along the facial nerve. In topographic-anatomic arrangement tumours from the brainstem down to the parotid gland are shown. The vestibulocochlear nerve and its related disorders fill the last chapter. The greatest part deals with diseases, especially tumours of the cerebellopontine angle. The central intra-axial parts of the acoustic pathway are also considered like lesions of the petrous apex affecting the vestibulocochlear nerve.

Drawing a conclusion, this book shows a very detailed and extensive description of CT and MRI findings of temporal bone diseases. We find a clear structure; disorders of adjacent regions are also regarded, especially in the posterior fossa and brainstem. CT and MRI scans show high-quality standard in technique and reproduction. Clear algorithms support the diagnostic procedure. A somewhat better connection between text and pictures and also technical data of the MR examinations would be desirable.

H. Stimmer, Munich

KARGER
Fax + 41 61 306 12 34
E-Mail karger@karger.ch
www.karger.com

© 1999 S. Karger AG, Basel

Accessible online at:
http://BioMedNet.com/karger

XLIX Temporal Bone Dissection Course

Barcelona, November 8–12, 1999

LXX Temporal Bone Dissection Course

Barcelona, March 2000

LXXI Temporal Bone Dissection Course

Barcelona, June 2000

A basically practical course dedicated to dissection. Surgery videos films and conferences.
Limited Places

Language: Spanish-Español

Information
Garcia-Ibañez Otologic Institute,
91, Dr. Roux St., 08017 Barcelona (Spain)
Tel. +34 93 205 02 04, Fax +34 93 205 43 67

XXVIII Course on Dissection and Microsurgery of the Paranasal Sinus

Barcelona, November 4–8, 1999

Films, videos and conferences.
Limited Places

Language: Spanish-Español

Information
Garcia-Ibañez Otologic Institute,
91, Dr. Roux St., 08017 Barcelona (Spain)
Tel. +34 93 205 02 04, Fax +34 93 205 43 67

NHS 2000: International Conference on Newborn Hearing Screening, Diagnosis and Intervention

Milan, October 12–14, 2000

Chairman: Ferdinando Grandori
Scientific Organizers: Ferdinando Grandori, Deborah Hayes

Important Dates
Abstract submission: May 15, 2000
Notification of acceptance: June 7, 2000
Registration and accommodation: June 30, 2000

Further details will be provided in winter 1999.

Registration Fees
300 EUROs (approx. US$ 330) before June 30, 2000
370 EUROs (approx. US$ 405) after June 30, 2000
Include: access to the scientific sessions, access to exhibits, books of conference abstracts, conference lunches and coffee-breaks, certificate of attendance.

Simultaneous translation to and from the most common languages shall be available if required by a sufficient number of participants.

Organizing Committee

In Milan:
Sharon Scagnetti, Paolo Ravazzani, Gabriella Tognola
Tel. +39 02 2399 3345/3344, Fax +39 02 2399 3367/3360
E-Mail NHS2000@biomed.polimi.it

In Denver:
Susan Dreith, Lisa Rider, Rebecca Mervine
Tel. +1 (303) 861 6800, Fax +1 (303) 764 8220

Information
In Europe, contact:
Dr. Ferdinando Grandori
Center of Biomedical Engineering
Polytechnic of Milan
Piazza Leonardo da Vinci 32
I–20133 Milan (Italy)
Fax +39 02 2399 3367, E-Mail NHS2000@biomed.polimi.it

In the USA, contact:
Dr. Deborah Hayes
Children's Hospital
1056 East 19th Ave., B030, Denver, CO 80218 (USA)
Tel. +1 (303) 861 6424, Fax +1 (303) 764 8220
E-Mail Hayes.deborah@tchden.org

KARGER
Fax + 41 61 306 12 34
E-Mail karger@karger.ch
www.karger.com

© 1999 S. Karger AG, Basel

Accessible online at:
http://BioMedNet.com/karger